& WELL® DIET:

The Higher Calorie Approach to Lifelong Weight Control and Good Nutrition

Diane M. Jouganatos, R.D., M.P.H.

BANTAM BOOKS

TORONTO • NEW YORK • LONDON • SYDNEY • AUCKLAND

This book is not intended to replace
your own physician with whom you should
consult before taking any medication or
considering treatment.

ALIVE & WELL® DIET
A Bantam Book / June 1984

ALIVE AND WELL® *and its letter device
are registered trademarks of Bristol-Myers
Company. Registered in U.S. Patent and Trademark
Office and elsewhere.*

ISBN 0-553-24117-6

Published simultaneously in the United States and Canada

---

*Bantam Books are published by Bantam Books, Inc. Its trade-
mark, consisting of the words "Bantam Books" and the por-
trayal of a rooster, is Registered in U.S. Patent and Trademark
Office and in other countries. Marca Registrada. Bantam
Books, Inc., 666 Fifth Avenue, New York, New York 10103.*

PRINTED IN THE UNITED STATES OF AMERICA

H   0 9 8 7 6 5 4 3 2 1

Acknowledgments

I would like to express my appreciation to my parents for their encouragement, to my sister for her patient assistance, to my brother for his editorial skills, to Solomon Delgado for his culinary expertise, and to Jim Thompson who made it all possible.

Contents

1 / A Higher Calorie Plan for Weight Loss

Chances are, if you are reading this book, this is not the first diet you have started. But, up until now, you may have thought that the fewer calories on the diet the better. This is not necessarily so, as you will see. In fact, low calorie diets can be counterproductive. Let me explain.

The *biggest* problem that the potential weight reducer faces is not weight reduction! By following any of the large number of diets currently in fashion, many people have achieved weight loss. The real problem is the ability to maintain weight, once reduction has been achieved. The dismal statistics are that fewer than ten percent of those who were successful in weight reduction will keep that weight off after five years. For the majority, the situation is one of on diet again, off diet again. I'm not suggesting that getting the weight off is that easy, but compared to the success rate in keeping the weight off, it is.

How is this so? When an individual starts on a diet, it most likely is an extremely strict and rigid diet, limited not only in the quantity of food, but in the quality of food. Usually, few foods are permitted on the diet, and individual selection and variety is minimal. As a result, the dieter is removing himself from temptations and palatabilities associated with the usual way in which he eats. With a limited selection of food and few choices to be made on the diet, the dieter is no longer experiencing eating as he had formerly, or as he probably will after he has reached his weight goal. There has been much publicity and popularity recently with liquid formula diets. The reason why these liquid diets work so well in achieving weight loss is that the formula diet takes away from the dieter the responsibility to select the proper food and to count calories. The dieter has a precalculated and premetered device for which the exact caloric value is known without his having to go through the effort of weighing and measuring portion size. The dieter does not have to select foods while on this liquid diet. Foods that were normally too tempting to keep to small or moderate portion size just aren't present in the formula diets. This phenomenon is not limited to formula diets but to any diet which severely restricts selection. The high protein, high fat diets such as the Atkins Diet, is such a situation. The dangerous fruit diet, recently appearing as the Beverly Hills Diet, is in the same category. So while some of these dietary regimens lead to weight loss, more often than not, it is not a permanent loss. Once the diet is stopped, the weight returns. A diet needs to be an instructive, educational process. It must provide the opportunity for practice in the desired behavior—namely proper food selection. Unfortunately, few diets prepare the individual for eating once the weight loss has been achieved. Most people return to old unhealthful styles of eating and cooking. Without the knowledge of basic nutrition concepts, without the practiced behavioral changes, and without an exercise program, the weight creeps back.

The diet issue is even more complex. Most "diets" are severely restricted in calories, ranging from 400 to 1,000 calories. Few people will stick to such diets for more than 6 or 8 weeks. These very low calorie diets should only be used by morbidly overweight individuals, and only under constant medical supervision. This is not always the case however, as very low calorie regimens are frequently used by individuals in the 20 to 30 pounds overweight range. These stringent diets are counterproductive in two ways. First, these diets are not instructive as to what "normal" eating habits are to be after the weight is lost, and these diets do not allow the dieter to practice the desired behavioral changes. In addition, very low calorie diets are counterproductive from a physiological viewpoint. It has been known for some time that there is a slowing of metabolic rate as caloric intake is reduced and as adaptation occurs to the new level of intake. The body adjusts to the low calorie diet so that even fewer calories are needed to produce a further weight loss. When the diet ends and the individual increases his calorie intake, weight is rapidly put back on. This occurs because the body's metabolic rate which was slowed during the period of caloric restriction, has not readjusted back to the higher, pre-diet rate. In effect, as a result of the very restricted diet, the body has adapted to require fewer calories. It appears that the chronic use of very low calorie diets can produce a permanently lowered metabolic rate. The lower the rate, the less food is required to *maintain* that weight.

Diets with moderate caloric restriction, such as the Alive and Well Diet, are less likely to produce metabolic compensation and have less danger of producing lasting metabolic changes. Furthermore, by using "real" food and healthful dietary practices, the Alive and Well Diet serves as a model for a lifetime of sound eating habits.

Most clinicians who work with overweight people report that weight lost slowly is more easily kept off. When a maximum of 2 to 3 pounds per week is lost, most of the loss is from fatty tissue. That is a desirable loss. That means that the yellowish-colored fat mass that may have accumulated inside your abdomen, upper arms, thighs, back, and so forth, is being "burned" off. When a weight loss faster than 2 or 3 pounds per week occurs, some lean, protein tissue is lost. This is undesirable. Lean tissue is muscle tissue. Muscle tissue is not expendable. It is needed to support our bodies in body movement and in vital organ function.

The Alive and Well Diet will provide you with the skills for selecting a well-balanced, lower calorie diet.

4 / ALIVE AND WELL DIET

The basic calorie level of the diet plan is 1,500 calories. The menus and recipes in this book will guide you in creating easy and delicious gourmet dishes which will provide you with the sensory pleasure that satisfies the appetite. The menus are precalculated to be 1,500 calories or less. They will help familiarize you with what you need to eat not only to lose weight, but to keep it off. The Alive and Well Diet plan is based on healthful, normal foods. The plan will instruct you on how to shop and select, cook, eat, and store food. These guidelines will not only benefit you, but benefit all those around you whose eating habits you can influence. For mothers, this means that the diet can serve as a preventative measure for children predisposed to overweight. In the coming chapters, we will be discussing the causes of overweight, how to calculate your rate of loss, basic nutrition and food composition, especially caloric composition, the incredible advantages of simple exercise, an effective psychological arsenal, and many more topics. I can assure you that if you follow along this book and if you earnestly desire to improve your body weight and health, you will succeed! The Alive and Well Diet is one of the most pleasurable but powerfully effective positive changes that you can make in your life.

2 / Overweight: Prevalence and Cause

Overweight is one of the most common of health problems. In fact, the prevalence of overweight has reached epidemic proportions in the United States. It is estimated that 50 to 80 million people in the United States are overweight. Excessive weight is considered by most as being unaesthetic and unattractive. For these reasons mostly, $10 billion are spent annually in various weight reduction treatments, ranging from diet food products, exercise gadgets, club memberships, records, manuals, and even body creams. However, aside from the unaesthetic qualities of being overweight, excess weight is associated with a reduced life span through the development of chronic health disorders such as heart and artery disease, high blood pressure, diabetes, gallbladder disease, and bone and joint disease. For many, being "fat" brings on real emotional disturbances. Achieving thinness becomes an obsession for many of us.

Why, then, are so many of us overweight? The answer is complex; but basically, excess weight results from an energy imbalance. That is when food (energy) is eaten in quantities that exceed the amount of energy the body uses in its normal repair and maintenance requirements and in our level of physical activity. We will maintain our present weight when the calories we consume equal the calories "burned" for normal tissue repair and for maintenance, in addition to the calories burned from any physical activity. In other words, maintaining a constant body weight can be represented by the following caloric balance equation:

Calories consumed = calories burned for maintenance and repairs + calories burned for physical activity.

When the amount of calories consumed exceeds that amount required for maintenance and for our level of physical activity, this equation becomes unbalanced. The equation now becomes:

Calories consumed = calories burned for maintenance and repairs + calories burned for physical activity + calories converted to fat storage.

This last equation represents what happens when we continuously consume more calories than we need. That is, we become overweight due to the accumulation of more and more fat.

From these equations, it can be seen that there are three major factors involved in the caloric balance equation. The first is the quantity and quality of food consumed. The second is the amount of calories (energy) our individual bodies use for routine body tissue repair and maintenance; for example, the formation of new blood cells; the constant relining of cells in the tissues of our digestive tracks; the formation of body proteins used as cell regulators; and the "running" of our heart, lungs, and brain while we are asleep. These functions, collectively called basal metabolism, are determined primarily by our heredity. The third and possibly the most important factor is physical activity.

Food habits directly influence the prevalence of

overweight. Our environment is perfectly suited for the development of overweight. For instance, as society becomes faster paced, as the percentage of women in the labor force increases, and as the importance attached to the use of leisure time increases, more meals are from convenience foods or eaten away from home. Unfortunately, these foods are often concentrated sources of calories and fat, as well as salt. The pattern of snacking coupled with the use of convenience foods, and eating away from home seems likely to continue in the United States. It is a hopeful sign that some eating establishments, as well as the convenience food industry, are introducing foods better suited for a health and weight conscious society. However, consumers need to be well informed to be able to make proper food selections given the enormity of the selections and the massive marketing and advertising of food items. Some advertising, whether deliberate or not, unfortunately misinforms the consumer. For example, many items which are advertised as being "dietetic" may simple be products in which the sugar has been replaced by a sugar substitute. The fat content may be identical to the non-"dietetic" counterpart. Total calories may also be very similar. Another example is the "diet plate" offered by some restaurants. In these diets, the starch has often been replaced by a serving of cottage cheese, and perhaps a slice of canned fruit. In actuality, the "diet plate" may be higher in fat and calories than the item it was substituting.

As previously discussed, part of the caloric balance equation involves our basal metabolism. There is some individual variation in the rate in which our bodies use calories for basal matabolism. This is called the basal metabolic rate, which is determined by our heredity to a large extent. Perhaps this factor accounts for the strong influence that familial traits exert on weight.

Studies that have been made with families of overweight persons have demonstrated that 40 percent of the children are overweight when one parent is overweight. If both parents are overweight, 80 percent of the children are overweight. Although parents are responsible in part for the eating habits of their children, statistics reveal that there are adopted children who are not overweight, even though their adoptive parents are. The age at which overweight first occurs influences the likelihood of overweight later on in adulthood. According to studies made in this area, if an individual is overweight before entering puberty, then the likelihood of ever being lean as an adult is approximately 25 percent. If the individual becomes overweight after puberty, then the chances of ever being lean as an adult are reduced to roughly 3 percent. This evidence points out the urgent need to start proper nutrition habits at a very early age as well as to incorporate physical activity into a daily routine from childhood on.

Physical activity is possibly the most important factor involved in weight maintenance. Physical activity can influence not only the rate at which our bodies use calories (energy) in maintenance, but also can influence the quantity of food that we consume. Studies have shown that for the proper control of food intake, there must be a certain amount of physical activity. The appetite control center of our brain can function properly only after a certain level of physical activity has been reached. In other words, after a program of exercise has been initiated, the body's appetite "thermostat" will be programmed to recognize satiety at a lower level of caloric intake. That is, you will feel like eating less. These studies lay to rest the notion that an increase in physical activity results in an increase in appetite. On the other hand, lumberjacks and others who have extremely high physical activity will, of course, require more calories and their appetite "thermostat" will read the appropriate cues.

Not only does physical activity assure the proper functioning of the brain's appetite control center, but it also pushes the caloric balance equation to favor weight loss while keeping the amount of food intake relatively unchanged. Children's weight can often be reduced simply by increasing their physical activity, without changing their food intake. Videotape studies of children engaged in various sports show that overweight children were less active participants than were the non-overweight children. The overweight children were, in effect, conserving energy and burning fewer calories, than the more active children. The fact that many of us are less active and have more sedentary jobs than earlier in this century, accounts for some of the reasons why we are more overweight than our ancestors. The greatest influence that physical activity has on our weight is that exercise increases the rate at which our bodies burn calories.

In summary, our physical inactivity, our reliance on convenience foods or eating out, and the availability of snack foods are all contributing factors to our overweight problem. No wonder 25 percent of us have a weight problem. For adult women over 30 years of age, 50 percent have a weight 10 percent greater than the ideal weight. For adult men over 30 years of age, 40 percent have a weight 10 percent greater than the ideal weight. The achievement and maintenance of the ideal weight is even harder for those with a family history of overweight, and for those who have been overweight as children and teenagers. Is it futile, then, to try to reduce in weight? Not at all! You can and will do it! But any program geared for weight reduction has to incorporate a new and better way of thinking about, and using, food. The plan must be sustainable over a lifetime. The Alive and Well Diet is such a plan. It stresses an increased knowledge of nutrition and the restructuring of old eating, cooking, shopping, and exercise patterns.

Now that you are aware of some of the causes and problems associated with overweight, let's turn to specifics about your ideal weight and the optimal rate of weight loss.

3 / Losing Weight

Defining "Overweight"

Overweight can be defined as weight in excess of that necessary for optimal body function. Scientists distinguish the difference between obesity and overweight as the former being the accumulation of excess fat, and the latter as being the weight above the average for a particular height and body type. The extra weight that an overweight person carries may be fat or lean tissue. An active professional football player may weigh more than the average for his height, but his weight is due to a large amount of muscle, which is lean tissue, and which is not in itself harmful. The same weight on a physically inactive man who holds a desk job, for example, would be the result of excessive fat tissue. It is this type of overweight that concerns us—excessive fat stores on our body. For the most part, this type of overweight is by far the most common. Therefore, when we will be speaking of overweight, from now on, we will be referring to the condition scientists refer to as obesity, or excessive fat accumulation.

Although definitions of overweight are imprecise,

there are several ways to assess overweight. The first is by simple observation; the second is the measurement of skinfold thickness, and the third is the comparison of weight with a standard weight for a particular height. The most obvious way to assess overweight is the visual observation of an unclothed individual. Is there a potbelly, flabby arms and legs, or rippling fat bulges over the back? As a rough estimate of overweight, this method is the easiest, although the least precise. Precision requires measurement. The second method of assessing overweight uses a measurement of skinfold thickness. The "pinch" test, in which you pinch yourself for an estimate of the thickness of the fat underneath the skin, is a simple version of the skinfold thickness measurement taken with standardized calipers. The skinfold thickness method of assessing overweight is based on the observation that excessive fat tissues are stored beneath the skin in overweight individuals. Skinfold calipers measure skinfold thickness at several body sites to give an average of body fat composition. Your percentage of body fat is then compared with the "desirable" percentage of body fat, which incidentally, may not be the average percentage of body fat in the population. For adult women, 22 percent of the body weight as fat is considered desirable; body fat greater than 30 percent is considered excessive. Whereas, for adult men, 15 percent of the body weight as fat is desirable, and greater than 20 percent is considered excessive. The greater allowance of fat for women is because women require more "essential" fat in their bodies than men, and because our culture conveys the notion that beauty is equated with a rounded figure.

The role that the "essential" fat stores plays for women is not entirely clear, but it is related to a protective mechanism for future childbearing. Very slender female runners and gymnasts who have a very low percentage of body fat, 5 to 10 percent, frequently stop menstruating temporarily. The relationship between body fat and female hormones is nature's way of reducing the chances for pregnancy to occur while the extra fat stores and the reserve energy supply in the form of fat, essential for pregnancy and subsequent nursing, are at a low level. Very active men, such as football players, runners, and others engaged in prolonged and intense physical exercise, may have fat stores approaching 5 percent. As we shall discuss later on, exercise facilitates the conversion of fat to lean muscle tissue. Body fat, and total body weight should not increase with age once adulthood is reached. That is, ideally, your weight and body fat at 55 years should not be more than what it was at 25 years, if at 25 you were at desirable levels of weight and body fat. Unfortunately, this is not what actually happens. Studies show that up to the age of 60 years, both men and women gain extra weight, which we call fat.

Finally, the most common method of assessing your overweight is to compare your weight with a standard. Standard weights for height, age, and sex have been developed; perhaps the most widely used is the Metropolitan Life Insurance Company's tables. However, these tables have their limitations. The tables list "average" weights of policyholders, which may not always be the ideal or desirable weight; furthermore, the weights listed do not distinguish between fat and muscle weight. On the other hand, these tables reflect the weights of people who have the greatest longevity and, presumably, the best health. Ideally, in determining optimal weight, other factors need consideration. These are body type, physical activity, distribution of weight over the body, and family history. Body type may play a greater role in determining our eventual weight and longevity than previously anticipated. Physical anthropologists have used a method of characterization of body type and shape based on muscle distribution and skeletal size as well as on weight. The three categorizations include ectomorphic, endomorphic, and mesomorphic body types. Ectomorphs are characterized by narrow and elongated extremities with slender skeletons and slender muscle mass. At the other end, endomorphs are characterized by large skeletons and large muscle mass. Mesomorphs fall somewhere in between these categorizations with moderate-size muscle mass and skeletons. For the most part, body type is determined at birth. Skeletal size cannot be changed, and muscle mass can be altered only to a degree by physical activity or inactivity. In a study of overweight adolescent girls, it was found that the overweight girls were primarily of the endomorphic type, with large muscles and skeletons, despite the girls' extreme inactivity. Very few ectomorphs were among the overweight girls. Moreover, in the adult population, the overweight are generally more endomorphic and mesomorphic and less ectomorphic than the nonoverweight. As we mentioned in the first chapter, there is a strong familial tendency toward overweight. Perhaps it is the inheritance of our body type that later on influences our weight.

The following height and weight table is a guide in identifying your ideal weight. Bear in mind that your level of activity, body type and composition, and family history must be taken into consideration when determining your ideal weight.

IDEAL BODY WEIGHT (IBW)

Height	Inches	IBW WOMEN Pounds	IBW MEN Pounds
5'0"	60	100	106
5'1"	61	105	112
5'2"	62	110	118
5'3"	63	115	124
5'4"	64	120	130
5'5"	65	125	136
5'6"	66	130	142
5'7"	67	135	148
5'8"	68	140	154
5'9"	69	145	160
5'10"	70	150	166
5'11"	71	155	172
6'0"	72	160	178
6'1"	73	165	184
6'2"	74	...	190
6'3"	75	...	196
6'4"	76	...	202
6'5"	77	...	208

IDEAL BODY WEIGHT (IBW)

Height	Inches	IBW WOMEN Pounds	IBW MEN Pounds
6'6"	78	...	214
6'7"	79	...	220
6'8"	80	...	226

CALCULATION OF IDEAL BODY WEIGHT

Women—100 pounds for first 5 feet, 5 pounds for each additional inch. Men—106 pounds for first 5 feet, 6 pounds for each additional inch. Add 10 percent for large frame; deduct 10 percent for small frame.

Now, if you have determined that you exceed your optimal weight, how do you go about reducing? Back to our earlier equation, excess weight occurs when more calories are consumed than are used (burned) as energy by the body. Weight maintenance occurs when

Calories consumed = calories burned for maintenance and repair + calories burned for physical activity or when $A = B + C$.

Weight gain occurs when A is larger than $B + C$. Weight loss occurs when $B + C$, the energy-consuming part of the equation, is larger than A, the calories consumed. So, by making either B or C larger, without changing A, the calories or food consumed, weight loss can be achieved. B, the calories, or energy, used in normal maintenance and repair, is for the most part, unchangeable. It is known as the basal metabolic rate, or BMR. The BMR is the minimum amount of calories, in the form of energy, that your body needs when you are at complete physical, mental, and emotional rest. You are most nearly at basal condition when you first awake in the morning. There is some individual variety in BMR levels, but not as wide as popularly believed. When you are ill with a fever, when you have broken a bone, or have had surgery, your BMR increases. An increase in physical activity can also indirectly increase your BMR. Many studies have shown that when subjects exercised, not only were calories expended during the exercise, but even 24 hours later the BMR was elevated by 10 to 15 percent. These results show that the benefits of exercise in weight loss appear to be greater than that resulting during the time of exercise alone. In other words, while you are sleeping after a day of exercise, your body is still burning calories at a faster pace than if you had not been exercising. Conversely, there is another situation in which your BMR can be reduced. When you start on a reducing diet, your body adapts to the lowered caloric intake by decreasing your BMR. This self-preservation mechanism comes into effect so that the body can ration out the available food energy and go further on fewer calories. This great ability of the body to adjust for survival can be a source of great frustration to the dieter. The less he eats, the less he needs to eat. Furthermore, total fasting reduces the BMR even more. The best solution, therefore, for anyone who desires to lose weight, is to combine a program of exercise with a diet which does not severely restrict caloric intake. The Alive and Well Diet is based on a 1,500-calorie plan, and on a daily exercise program which includes at least 30 minutes of moderately vigorous activity per day. The diet plan can be modified to total 1,200 calories for those who are physically unable to exercise, or for those who require fewer calories to reduce in weight. With this total diet and exercise program, we can assure that all three parts of the original equation, $A = B + C$, where A is the total caloric intake, B is the BMR (calories for maintenance and repair), and C is calories in the form of energy for usage during physical activity, will be changed at the same time, in favor of weight loss.

Calculating the Rate of Weight Loss

The weight that you want to lose will be mostly from fatty tissue. Fatty tissue is associated with water in the body, and therefore, some weight loss will be from water loss. Most medical authorities are in agreement that a weight loss of no greater than 2 or 3 pounds per week is safe and generally does not require medical supervision. At a loss of 2 pounds per week, you'll be losing mostly fat. At a faster rate of weight loss, protein tissue, such as muscle will be lost, in addition to water and some fat. If you are extremely overweight and there is a pressing indication for a more rapid weight loss, you should be under close and frequent medical supervision. The rate of weight loss can be predicted by the fact that one pound of fatty tissue is the caloric equivalent of about 3,500 calories. This means that if you incur a daily deficit of 500 calories, either by eating 500 calories less, or by increasing your daily activity by 500 calories, you will, after seven days, have incurred a deficit of 3,500 calories, and therefore, lost one pound of fat. Ideally, a decrease in food intake should be coupled with an increase in physical activity. For example, if you decrease your daily food consumption by 500 calories per day, and increase your physical activity by 500 calories per day, totaling 1,000 calories per day, after seven days you will have spent 7,000 calories, or two pounds of fat. To determine how quickly you will lose weight, you need to know how many calories your body requires to maintain your present weight.

To calculate this caloric requirement, the following guidelines are used by nutritionists:

Level of Activity	Calories Needed per Pound of Present Weight
Sedentary	13 – 14
Moderately active	15 – 17
Very active	18 +

You would be considered to be moderately active if you exercise for 30 minutes daily, and use your body in a range of motions throughout the day. A very active level of activity applies to those individuals who are engaged in sustained strenuous physical activity for the major part of the day. Sedentary applies to individuals who are generally in a resting physical condition for most of the day.

If you are moderately active and weigh 150 pounds, you require 150 x 15 or 2,250 calories per day to maintain your weight of 150 pounds. The 2,250 calories per day would keep your weight at 150 pounds if your level of activity remained the same. But let's say that you are 5 feet 4 inches in height and weigh 150 pounds; you consider yourself to be overweight by about 30 pounds. Your goal is to reach 120 pounds. When you start following the Alive and Well Diet 1,500-calorie plan, you will have a deficit of 750 calories per day:

$$
\begin{array}{rl}
2250 & \text{calories required to maintain 150 pounds} \\
-1500 & \text{calories in the Alive and Well Diet plan} \\
\hline
750 & \text{calories per day deficit}
\end{array}
$$

The 750 calories a day less than what you need will amount to 5,250 calories deficit in 7 days, which equals a loss of 1½ pounds of fat per week. If at the same time, you increase your activity, you will lose weight faster as the relative requirement for calories increases with exercise. By exercising daily, you could use up 250 to 500 calories more per day which would yield a weight loss of ½ to 1 pound or more per week. Furthermore, with exercise, the loss of lean muscle tissue is spared. With exercise, more fatty tissue is lost. If you add the weight loss from exercise to the weight loss from reduced caloric intake in this example, a total of about 3 pounds per week would be lost. In the first few days or even first few weeks of starting a new diet, some individuals experience a greater rate of weight loss as a result of a normal diuresis, or water loss from tissues in the body. The Alive and Well Diet also has a 1,200-calorie plan geared for individuals who are unable to exercise, or who for various reasons are unable to reduce in weight at a satisfactory rate on the 1,500-calorie plan. If you use the 1,200-calorie plan of the Alive and Well Diet, then you will have a deficit of 1,050 calories per day, assuming you weigh 150 pounds:

$$
\begin{array}{rl}
2,250 & \text{calories needed to maintain 150 pounds} \\
-1,200 & \text{calories in the Alive and Well Diet plan} \\
\hline
1,050 & \text{calories per day deficit}
\end{array}
$$

The 1,050-calorie deficit for 7 days yields a 7,350-calorie deficit at the end of the week, which represents about 2 pounds of fat loss, since 3,500 calories are in 1 pound of fat.

Again, adding water loss, usually 1 pound of water is lost for every 7 pounds of fat tissue, and weight loss as a result of possibly increased physical activity, the total weight loss becomes greater than 2 pounds. A weight loss greater than 3 pounds per week is associated with the loss of body muscle tissue. Excessive loss of muscle tissue is not desirable and not conducive to good health. There is evidence that shows that weight loss in very overweight individuals is achieved by more loss of body fat than of lean body tissue. Yet, in individuals at near optimal body weight, a lower calorie diet results in weight loss as a result of the loss of both fat and lean tissue. For this reason, very low calorie diets are not recommended except under very special circumstances. Severe restriction of calories in an individual who is 10 to 20 pounds overweight results mostly in the loss of muscle tissue. The heart is a muscle as are other vital body organs. The significance of protein loss from these muscle tissues, and whether the protein is replaced when calories become available is not known, yet.

The formula we have used to predict weight loss is theoretical, based on the calorie value of a pound of fat, and based on the average of the experience of weight loss in groups of people. As we mentioned earlier, water loss is associated with fat loss. In addition, some lean tissue, such as capillaries and muscle which were needed to support the fatty tissue, will also be lost. Few people experience as smooth a weight loss as would be predicted by the formula. Body tissues do not work that way. Usually, weight loss lags a bit behind the cutdown in food intake or increases in activity. By using the formulas we have described, you will be able to estimate your own weight loss. Remember that the starting point is first to calculate the calories you require to maintain your present weight. Subtract either 1,500 or 1,200 from this figure. Multiply this figure by 7 and, then, divide by 3,500 in order to figure how many pounds a week you will lose. This will be a rough estimate. Only in a laboratory could you determine with precision the calories that you require daily to maintain your present weight. The heavier you are, therefore, the more calories you need to maintain your weight, and the more pronounced the weight loss on the 1,500- or 1,200-calorie level. In addition, the heavier you are, the more effective your exercise program will be. You will burn more calories doing the same exercise or activity as a thinner person because you have the added burden of extra weight to move around. It takes more energy to move just as it would be if you were carrying weight while exercising. The best route to the achievement of optimal weight is to combine moderate food intake with a moderate exercise program.

Now, a very important point. The goal of the Alive and Well Diet is long-term weight loss. A slow and steady weight loss is the best. Gradual and persistent weight loss is superior to a fast and sudden loss. To lose 10 pounds in 5 weeks, as we recommend, is much better than losing 10 pounds in 2 weeks. Fast changes in weight are usually only temporary changes. A slow and persistent weight loss is most likely to be a permanent loss. Don't say you are an exception to the rule and if you could only lose 25 pounds in a month you'd keep it off. The odds are not in your favor I'm afraid. A weight loss of about 2 pounds per week is ideal and will greatly improve your chances for the biggest problem you face—permanent weight loss.

4 / Nutrition: Basic Definitions

The biggest roadblock on the way of sound eating habits and weight loss is nutritional misinformation. Books, magazine and newspaper articles, lectures by persons with questionable credentials, television talk shows, and advertisements of all kinds, bombard us with new "theories," breakthroughs, the latest diets which allegedly worked for so many, creams, wraps, pills, and dietary supplements. Undeniably, the consumer can be justifiably confused. So, before proceding further with a discussion on diet and nutrition, there needs to be an understanding of the basic elements of nutrition. Certain terms must be clarified. The most common will now be reviewed.

Diet refers to what a person usually eats and drinks. It is a broadly used word and often refers in common parlance to a weight reduction regimen. However, when I ask you to tell me about your diet, I am asking that you describe what you eat on a typical day.

A **calorie** is a unit of heat, like a degree Fahrenheit, but it is on a different scale. One calorie is the amount of heat that is required to raise the temperature of one gram of water from 14.5°C to 15.5°C. When food is broken down by the body to be used as fuel or repair material, energy is released. This energy produces heat. The calorie level of food is the measure of the amount of energy it provides to the body.

A **gram** is a unit of weight measurement. The gram system is used for all scientific work. It is also used by the Europeans in their daily living, as opposed to the system we use in the United States, ounces and pounds. It takes 28 grams to make one ounce. A kilo, abbreviation for kilogram, is worth 2.2 pounds.

Vitamins are organic substances occurring in small amounts in fresh foods such as plants and the flesh of animals. Most vitamins cannot be made by the body and therefore need to be consumed. Vitamins are required for the maintenance of normal metabolic function in the body. The absence of one or more vitamins in the diet would result in specific metabolic defects. The water soluble vitamins are vitamin C, folic acid, thiamin (B_1), riboflavin (B_2), niacin, B_6, B_{12}, biotin, and pantothenic acid. The fat-soluble vitamins are A, D, E, and K. There is no such thing as B_{15} or B_{17}.

Metabolism is the sum total of all the physical and chemical processes by which an organism such as man converts simpler compounds such as food, into living, organized substances such as cells and tissues, and then reconverts such material into simple compounds while releasing energy for its use. Taking simpler compounds such as food and converting them into organized substances like tissue, is called growth or maintenance. These organized tissues can be reconverted to simpler compounds for use as an energy source when no simpler compounds, such as food, are available. This process, if it continues, is the weight reduction process.

Minerals are nonorganic compounds which are essential to the body. They may be used as part of structural tissue, such as calcium and phosphorus in bones, or they may be part of an organic molecule such as iron in the hemoglobin molecule which is part of the red blood cell. Some minerals are essential to the body in trace amounts. These minerals usually serve as constituents of enzyme systems in the body, or as part of hormones, such as iodine. You may have heard of the trace minerals such as zinc, copper, manganese, fluoride, chromium, selenium, and molybdenum, to name a few.

Carbohydrates are a group of compounds which have a related structure. The arrangement of these atoms determines whether they are complex carbohydrates, called starches, or carbohydrates, called sugars. One gram of a carbohydrate is worth about 4 calories. Foods high in starch include breads, cereals, potatoes, and rice. Fruits and sweets of all kinds contain sugar. Glucose is the sugar our bodies use for energy. To a large extent, one of the reasons why we eat food is to provide our bodies with a source of glucose.

Proteins are a group of similar compounds, without which life could not be supported. All forms of life have protein as a constituent part. In the body, proteins act as structural features of the cell, as organic catalysts (enzymes), as messengers (hormones), and as antibodies. Protein in the diet is important primarily in that it is a source of *amino acids,* the building blocks of proteins. There are some nine essential amino acids that cannot be made in the body by precursors. Animal tissue, such as meat, eggs, and milk are high in protein content. Legumes, such as dried peas and beans are also good sources of protein. While grains contain a significant amount of protein, their amino acid makeup is such that some of the essential amino acids are present in very low quantities thereby making grains an incomplete protein source. For adults, protein requirements are set at about 0.35 grams per pound of weight. Thus, for a 154-pound man the protein requirement is around 56 grams of protein per day; for a woman weighing 120 pounds, the figure is about 42 grams per day. Infants and children have a relatively greater requirement for protein per pound of weight. The "typical" American adult diet provides around 80 to 90 grams of protein daily. One gram of protein provides approximately 4 calories.

Fats are a group of compounds of similar structure which are found in animals and plants. Fats are the most concentrated form of energy available to the body, providing 9 calories per gram of fat. Because of their concentrated nature, fats serve as energy stores in the body. Fats are mostly 16 to 18 carbon atoms strung together. When the carbon atoms are all attached to hydrogen atoms, the fat is saturated. When few of the carbon atoms are attached to hydrogen atoms, the fat is unsaturated. Common saturated fats are lard, coconut oil, palm oil, and butter. Common polyunsaturated fats are safflower oil, corn oil, cottonseed oil, and sunflower oil.

Cholesterol is a type of fat found in animal tissues only. Vegetable oils have no cholesterol. Cholesterol is an integral part of the cell structure and is synthesized in most of the tissues of the body. In fact, about 40 percent of the circulating cholesterol is derived from the diet, with the remaining being derived from that cholesterol which the body manufactures. High blood cholesterol levels are associated with plaque formation in the arteries. This condition is known as arteriosclerosis and is the leading cause of heart disease. Polyunsaturated fats tend to produce a decrease in blood cholesterol levels, while saturated fats tend to produce an increase.

Fiber, often referred to as roughage or bulk, describes those components of plant material which are not broken down by the enzymes in the human gastrointestinal tract. Most fiber is complex carbohydrate, but not all. Cellulose, hemicellulose, lignin, pectins, and guar gums are some common forms of fiber. Fiber does not supply nutrients to the body, although fiber is frequently associated with nutrient rich foods. Fiber provides bulk to the intestinal contents and has a water-absorbing property. This affects the proper function and health of the intestines and colon. Some types of fiber, particularly pectins and guar gums, can effect a lowering of blood cholesterol levels, and delay stomach-emptying time.

Organic refers to compounds manufactured by living things, plants and animals. The terms *organic, natural,* and *health* foods tend to be used interchangeably among promoters of these foods. There is little agreement on their exact meaning. However, *organic* foods or *organically grown* foods allegedly are grown without agricultural chemicals and are processed without chemicals or additives.

"Natural" foods are marketed as foods produced with minimal processing and without the use of additives or other artificial ingredients.

"Health" foods encompass both *natural* and *organic* foods, but the term *health* is supposed to connote that these foods have special health-promoting properties. There are no industry standards for *natural, organic,* and *health* foods. There is no evidence that these foods are safer, more nutritious, and somehow better for you.

Dietetic foods are prepared foods that are either lowered in salt or sugar content, or some other component, but are foods that are intended to be substitutes for commonly eaten foods, by those persons who are on special diets. "Dietetic" ice cream and candy bars are examples. Often, however, the substituted item, sugar for sorbital for example, does not change the calorie level of that food. Dietetic candy bars and cookies have as many calories as the "real thing." Careful label reading should preceed selection of these food items.

Additives are compounds added to food and generally fall into the following classes:

Antioxidants are used to prevent browning of fruits and rancidity of fats. Common antioxidants are BHA, BHT, tocopherols (vitamin E derivatives), ascorbic acid (vitamin C), and citric acid.

Preservatives are used to control the growth of bacteria, yeast, and mold. The most common are sodium benzoate, calcium propionate (occurs naturally in Swiss cheese), propionic acid, potassium sorbate, and sulfur dioxide.

Emulsifiers are used to blend liquids together for more uniform consistency and texture. Examples include lecithin and mono and diglycerides.

Stabilizers and thickeners are used to maintain

uniform color, flavor, and texture. Common examples include agar, cellulose, guar gums, gelatin, pectin, and dextrin.

Sodium nitrite is used to inhibit the growth of botulism organisms and is added to cured meats. Nitrites may react with amines in protein rich foods to produce nitrosamines, potential carcinogens in laboratory animals. Vitamin C inhibits nitrosamine production.

Coloring agents and **flavoring agents** may be natural or synthetic. Other miscellaneous additives include anticaking and antifoaming agents, flavor enhancers (for example, monosodium glutamate, or MSG), and various firming and bleaching agents.

Nutritive additives include vitamins and minerals which have been added to foods.

Fortification means that nutrients are added in amounts that exceed the levels ordinarily found in the food. *Enrichment* refers to the addition of certain nutrients to grains.

Processed refers to any steps taken in the chain of events from when a food source is picked off a plant or animal, to when it reaches the consumer. Raw fruits are virtually unprocessed. TV dinners are completely processed foods, or *convenience*.

Enzymes are complex organic compounds secreted by living cells which are capable of causing or accelerating changes in specific substances. Enzymes are destroyed by heat and acid. There is no evidence that the ingestion of enzymes in other than medically indicated situations serves a useful purpose.

5 / Rationale of the Alive and Well Diet

A Diet for Good Health

First and foremost, a diet should promote and maintain good health. The Alive and Well Diet is such a diet in addition to promoting a weight loss. It is based on well-accepted nutritional guidelines which are advocated by scientific and government bodies such as the Department of Agriculture, the Department of Health and Human Services, the surgeon general, the Senate Select Committee on Nutrition and Human Needs, and the American Heart Association.

The following dietary guidelines form the basis of the Alive and Well Diet:

1. Achievement and maintenance of ideal body weight is very desirable for overall good health.
2. A wide variety of foods should be eaten daily to assure that nutrients are consumed in necessary quantities.
3. Intake of fat should be reduced in total to about thirty percent of the total calories consumed.

4. Intake of sodium should be moderated.
5. Adequate consumption of fresh fruits, vegetables, and whole grains rich in fiber should be ensured, while the consumption of sugar should be reduced.

It is important to note that these guidelines are intended for the general public. Some individuals may have been prescribed different dietary guidelines by their doctors for special medical conditions. But for the great majority of the U.S. public, these dietary guidelines form the basis of a life-style that will help to reduce the risk of heart disease, diabetes, high blood pressure, and possibly some cancers. In addition, these dietary guidelines help to reduce the risk of being overweight and form the basis of a weight reduction diet for overweight persons. Now we will take up each of the guidelines.

1. Achievement and maintenance of ideal weight is very desirable for overall good health.

Overweight presents both physical and psychological disturbances. Overweight places a stress on major bodily functions. High blood pressure is more prevalent among overweight persons. Overweight persons with elevated blood pressure show a greater rate of illness and death from coronary heart disease than nonoverweight persons with high blood pressure. Very overweight persons may have greater difficulty in normal breathing due to the additional weight carried on the chest wall. This leads to a diminished exercise tolerance. Cardiac enlargement and poor resistance to even mild respiratory infections may also result from extreme overweight. There is a high prevalence of impaired glucose (blood sugar) tolerance and elevated blood sugar levels among overweight individuals. There is a significant association between overweight and gallbladder disease. Being overweight tends to aggravate a number of bone and joint diseases when the extra weight places pressure on the damaged areas. Overweight persons are at an increased risk of developing complications during and following surgery. Overweight persons are faced with social problems as well. There is a tendency for overweight persons to be discriminated against with respect to employment and promotions. Studies have indicated that overweight people are frequently perceived as having emotional problems that result in overweight, as being indifferent to their own appearance, as well as totally lacking in self-control. An obsessive concern with self-image, and often, especially in younger people, passivity and social withdrawal, compound the problem. Many of these psychological effects of being overweight tend to make the condition self-perpetuating. When dieting is attempted, it is usually an extreme change from normal eating patterns, and does not lead to long-term good diet habits and weight control. A cycle of losing and regaining excess weight evolves. Not surprisingly, anxiety, irritability, and depression frequently follow.

2. A wide variety of foods should be eaten daily to assure that nutrients are consumed in necessary quantities.

The human body requires a wide assortment of nutrients to survive and to maintain health. These include the vitamins, minerals, amino acids which are the building blocks of proteins, fatty acids, and of course water. Certain foods are better sources of some of the nutrients than others. Therefore, to assure an adequate supply of nutrients, we need to eat from a wide variety of foods on a daily basis. To simplify our daily meal selection, the Department of Agriculture devised in 1954, a practical system of food categorization known as the Four Food Groups.

THE FOUR FOOD GROUPS

Group	Major Nutrients
I. Milk group	Calcium Protein Riboflavin (B$_2$)

THE FOUR FOOD GROUPS

Group	Major Nutrients
II. Meat or Meat alternate group	Protein Iron Niacin Thiamin (B_1)
III. Fruit/vegetable group	Vitamin A Vitamin C
IV. Bread/cereal group	Carbohydrate Thiamin Iron Niacin

By consuming the suggested minimum number of servings from each group that is recommended for persons of various stages of life, an adequate supply of essential nutrients is possible.

SUGGESTED SERVINGS FROM EACH FOOD GROUP

	Adults	Adolescents	Infants and Children	Pregnancy/ Lactation
I. Milk group	2	4	3	4
II. Meat or Meat alternate group	2	2	2	3
III. Fruit/vegetable group	4	4	4	4
IV. Bread/cereal group	4	4	4	4

FOODS AND SERVINGS SIZES

Group	One Serving Size
I. Milk group	8 oz milk or yogurt 1½ oz cheese 2 c cottage cheese
II. Meat or Meat Alternate group	2 oz cooked meat, fish, or poultry 2 eggs 1 c cooked dry beans or peas ½ c nuts or seeds
III. Fruit/vegetable group	½ c cooked fruit or vegetable 1 c raw whole fruit
IV. Bread/cereal group	1 slice bread ½ c cooked rice, pasta, or cereal

The Basic Four Food Groups were developed as a system which translated the Recommended Dietary Allowances (RDA) into actual food-related information which would be understandable to the public. The RDAs are the levels of intake of essential nutrients considered by the Food and Nutrition Board of the National Research Council to be adequate to meet known nutritional needs of practically all healthy persons. You might find the RDA for several nutrients on food package labels. RDAs also vary with various stages of life. The "USRDA" on your cereal box refers to the recommended allowance for a specific nutrient for the adult male as a group. The Basic Four-Food Group system allows you to judge the adequacy of any diet. When you see or hear about a new diet, or even one that has been around for a while, compare it to the Basic Four. If it falls below in some or all of the food groups, chances are good that it is not nutritionally adequate.

The Alive and Well Diet also uses a categorization of foods into groups with similar composition. We have expanded the Basic Four into a "Basic Six." The additional groups have been made to reflect the calorie differences between fruits and vegetables, so that now two groups exist where one had in the Basic Four, and to include the fats into a separate group. The Basic Six Food Groups will be discussed at length in the next chapter. The Alive and Well Diet provides the RDA for the major nutrients for most healthy people.

3. Intake of fat should be reduced in total to about thirty percent of the total calories consumed.

Heart disease is a major cause of death and disability in the United States. High blood cholesterol levels are associated with heart disease. Populations such as the United States with diets high in saturated fats and cholesterol, tend to have high blood cholesterol levels. There are, however, inherent differences among individuals in their regulation of blood cholesterol levels, and in their responses to dietary cholesterol. In addition to genetic factors, environmental factors such as exercise, alcohol intake, and dietary components such as total calories, fiber, and total fat seem to affect blood levels of cholesterol. While there is controversy about recommendations to alter intakes of fat and cholesterol for the general public, recommendations to reduce dietary fat are indeed sensible. There are more reasons than blood cholesterol to reduce total fat intake. The "average" American diet is approximately 40- to 45-percent fat calories. Fats are a concentrated source of calories, more than double in calories compared with carbohydrates or proteins. As a result, a diet high in fat will also be high in calories. Lowering the fat intake daily to no more than 30 percent of total calories will provide a greater intake of less calorically dense foods, and will automatically lower caloric intake. When foods such as fruits and vegetables and whole grain products are eaten in place of fats, the diet becomes richer in vitamins, minerals, and fiber. Oils, margarine, butter, and mayonnaise are almost entirely fats and should be limited to a small quantity daily. Salad dressings and fatty meats such as bacon, sausage, cold cuts, and marbled meats are also high in fat and are to be avoided. Whole milk and cheese, while rich in many nutrients, also contain fat and therefore lower fat milks and cheeses are preferred on a diet. Pastry such as pies, cookies, and cakes are high in fat as well as sugar. However, it is possible to bake delicious cakes, pies, and cookies which are low fat and low sugar, as you will see in our Alive and Well recipes.

4. Intake of sodium should be moderated.

Approximately 18 percent of American adults have high blood pressure, a major risk factor for coronary heart disease, strokes, blood vessel disease, and chronic kidney disease. Although the causes of high blood pressure are still undefined for 90 percent of those with this disorder, there appears to be both genetic and environmental influences. Epidemiological studies (studies to find the cause of a particular condition) have suggested that in countries and regions where there is a high sodium intake there is a higher incidence of high blood pressure. In societies where sodium intake is very low, high blood pressure is virtually unknown. Studies with laboratory animals have shown that certain sodium sensitive strains of laboratory animals whose pressure is normal on a low sodium diet have elevations of blood pressure when they were fed a high sodium diet. The same breed of animal, but not of the sodium sensitive strain, demonstrated no change in blood pressure with the higher intake of sodium. It is believed that certain people are also genetically susceptible to high blood pressure. It is for this group of people for whom high sodium intake poses a greater health risk. Because there is no definitive way at present to predict who will develop high blood pressure, a lower sodium diet might help potentially susceptible individuals from developing the condition. Recently, research has reexamined the dietary factors that may contribute to high blood pressure. Interest has been generated from studies that suggest that low potassium intake (an element abundant in many fruits and vegetables) may contribute to high blood pressure. Relatively new studies suggest that calcium may also be an important factor in blood pressure regulation. Again, epidemiological studies, experimental animal studies, and human dietary surveys seem to indicate that a low calcium intake is associated with high blood pressure.

Until all the evidence is in, it is a prudent measure for most of us to be moderate in our sodium intake. The Alive and Well Diet uses salt sparingly in its menus and recipes. The diet also provides at least the Recommended Dietary Allowance for calcium, if not more. The potassium level in the diet is high due to the inclusion of four fruits per day and many vegetables.

5. Adequate consumption of fresh fruits, vegetables, and whole grains rich in fiber should be insured, while the consumption of sugar should be reduced.

The consumption of fruits and vegetables in the United States has declined throughout this century. More and more fat and protein foods displace the fruits and vegetables and whole grains once consumed. Fruits and vegetables and whole grains are rich in carbohydrates, vitamins, minerals, and fiber. In particular, fruits and vegetables are sources of vitamins A and C. Recently, the National Research Council Committee on Diet, Nutrition, and Cancer suggested that Americans should increase their consumption of fruits and vegetables that are high in vitamin C, such as citrus fruits, and beta-carotene (the previtamin A that the body can convert into the vitamin itself) such as dark green and deep yellow or orange vegetables. The committee has based these suggestions on evidence that increased intakes of vitamin C and beta-carotene may be associated with a reduced risk of some cancers. The same committee also recommended a reduction in total dietary fat to 30 percent of total calories. Fruits and vegetables contain almost no fat and are a rich source of fiber. A diet high in fibrous foods leads to a more rapid passage of foods through the intestinal tract. This results in bulkier and more frequent bowel movements and relief from constipation. Diets which are high in fiber, especially those high in pectin, which is found in fruit, have the benefit of lowering blood cholesterol levels. It is believed that this occurs by the following mechanism. In the body, the liver uses cholesterol to make bile acids which are secreted into the intestine to aid in digestion.

Some bile acids are reabsorbed from the intestines and recycled, or conserved, to be used again. When adequate fiber is consumed, some of it binds the bile acids and allows them to be excreted by the body. The liver has to then draw upon its cholesterol reserves in order to replenish the bile acids. As a result, the body's cholesterol reserves are used up faster. It has also been proposed that a high fiber diet may reduce the risks of colon cancer. By its association with water in the intestines, fiber in the diet tends to dilute the contents of the intestines. Potentially irritating and possibly cancer-causing substances in the intestines and colon are thereby reduced in potency. In addition, a diet high in fiber from fruits and vegetables and whole grains is useful in weight reduction as the fiber seems to promote satiety and reduce hunger. The reasons for this are that fiber in the diet provides bulk which results in a feeling of fullness sooner and also, some types of fiber especially pectin and guar, cause a delay in the stomach emptying which also gives a feeling of satiety.

Whole grain products such as whole wheat bread, brown rice, oats, whole wheat cereals, and corn, are rich sources of the vitamins thiamin and niacin. Whole grain products are mostly carbohydrate, starch in particular, and contain very little fat, but significant amounts of protein. Protein content ranges from 10 to 14 percent compared to about 22 percent for legumes such as dried beans and peas, and 18 percent for lean meats.

Some vegetables such as potatoes and dried beans are high in starch content. Other vegetables, particularly green vegetables, are low in starch and high in water content, therefore low in calories. Fruits also contain carbohydrates, in particular the sugar, fructose. White or brown granulated sugar and honey are refined sugars which are devoid of vitamins, minerals, protein, or fiber. As a source only of calories (and taste), refined sugars should be avoided. Many Americans have the misconceived notion that carbohydrates, especially starch, are fattening and therefore to be avoided in a diet. In fact, the intake of starch should be increased in most people in proportion to the fat and protein levels of the diet. Carbohydrates in the diet should be at least 50 percent of the total calories consumed. Fat as we mentioned earlier, should be no greater than 30 percent of the total calories consumed. The "typical" American diet is about 45 percent fat. The remaining 20 percent should be from protein, although an intake of 12 to 15 percent of the total calories in the diet from protein is sufficient for most people. The Alive and Well Diet is based on a carbohydrate, protein, and fat distribution of 50 percent, 20 percent, and 30 percent of total calorie intake, respectively.

A Diet for Weight Reduction and Weight Maintenance

The Alive and Well diet, as we have been discussing all along, is not only a health-promoting diet, but also a diet for weight loss. It is a diet which teaches you what you should eat and how you should prepare foods, even after you have reached your ideal weight. The best part is that you will not feel deprived or punished. A glance at the menus and recipes will convince you of that. Because the Alive and Well Diet plan is a relatively high-caloried reduction plan, it will not induce undesirable counterproductive changes in your metabolic rate. As discussed earlier, lower calorie diets tend to decrease your body's metabolic rate, the rate your body uses calories. As a result, your body will adapt and require fewer calories. This life-preserving adaptive mechanism is great if you are caught in the mountains during a blizzard and food is unavailable, or if you are stranded on a raft in the middle of the ocean without food. But most of us do not need this adaptation, for chronic lowering of the metabolic rate can result in a permanent reduction in the metabolic rate, thereby a permanent reduction in the amount of food we can eat. Now let's turn to specifics about the actual food on the diet plan.

6 / Composition of the Basic Diet Plan

Once you become familiar with and practice the Alive and Well Diet, you will have in your possession a valuable tool which will aid you in reducing and staying reduced for good. The diet plan is intended to be instructive. There will be some things that you must learn. Be wary of advertisements for reducing diet plans which claim that you don't have to *learn* or *think* about anything. If "they" have done all the thinking for you and all you have to do is follow their plan, what do you have that you can use once you are at desired weight and want to stay at that weight? Any wonder why the statistics for the maintenance of weight after reduction are so distressingly poor?

You need to be knowledgeable about what you are preparing to eat. The Alive and Well Diet will familiarize you with a system of food categorization and portioning which is used by professional dietitians and nutritionists. This system will allow you to quickly assess the calorie value of most foods. By using this system you can make intelligent, informed food selections which will assure you of a nutritious, healthful diet. After all, we desire to be slim and trim for the sake of our appearance. Appearance also includes smooth skin, shiny hair, good teeth and nails, and robust health and energy. A nutritious diet will maximize your looks. With the Alive and Well Diet you will be able to adjust the diet plan for more or less rapid weight loss, or for weight maintenance. Best of all, you will be able to incorporate all of your favorite foods into the diet. By adjusting your recipes in certain ways, you will have transformed formerly high calorie dishes into a lowered calorie, more healthful cuisine.

The basic diet plan is formulated around six basic food groups. Foods are grouped together based on the similar nutrients they contain. For example, foods high in protein and calcium make up the *milk* group. Foods which are primarily fat in content make up the *fat* group. Foods which are primarily starches make up the *starch* group, and so forth. These are the six groups:

1. Fruit group
2. Starch group
3. Meat group
4. Fat group
5. Milk group
6. Vegetable group

Within each group, foods are listed in specific quantities. These quantities are the "units," and every unit within the same group will be the same in calorie value. For example, in the fruit unit group, ½ cup of orange juice is equal in calorie value with ¾ cup of strawberries, or 2 tablespoons of raisins, or 1 medium peach. When your diet plan calls for one fruit unit, you may select any food within the fruit group but only in the quantity listed. The following are the 6 food groups:

FRUIT UNIT GROUP*

Apples	1 med	Bananas	½ small
Apple juice	⅓ c	Blackberries	½ c
Applesauce	½ c	Blueberries	½ c
Apricots, fresh	2 med	Boysenberries	½ c
Apricots, dried	4 halves	Cantaloupes	¼ small
Apricot nectar	⅓ c	Cherries	10 large

FRUIT UNIT GROUP*

Cranberry juice	¼ c	Peaches	1 med
Dates	2	Peach nectar	⅓ c
Figs, fresh	1	Pears	1 med
Figs, dried	1	Pear nectar	⅓ c
Fruit cocktail	½ c	Persimmons	1 small
Grapefruit	½	Pineapple cubes	½ c
Grapefruit sections	½ c	Pineapple rings	2
Grapefruit juice	½ c	Pineapple juice	⅓ c
Grapes	12	Plums	2 med
Grapes, seedless	12	Pomegranates	⅓ med
Grape juice	¼ c	Prunes	2 med
Guava	1 med	Prune juice	¼ c
Honeydew melon	⅛ med	Raisins	2 tbsp
Kumquats	4 med	Raspberries	½ c
Lemon juice	¾ c	Rhubarb, raw, cubes	1 c
Lime juice	¾ c	Strawberries	¾ c
Loganberries	½ c	Tangelos	1 med
Mangoes	½ med	Tangerines	1 med
Nectarines	1 med	Watermelon cubes	1 c or ½ slice, 10″ x ¾″ thick
Oranges	1 med		
Orange sections	½ c		
Orange juice	½ c		
Papayas	⅓ med		

*All fruit is fresh or canned in water or unsweetened juice.
1 fruit unit = 50 calories, 12 grams carbohydrate, 0 grams protein, and 0 grams fat.

STARCH UNIT GROUP

*Breads**

White (including French and Italian)	1 slice
Whole wheat	1 slice
Sourdough, wide loaf	½ slice
Rye or pumpernickel	1 slice
Raisin	1 slice
Bagel, small	½
†Biscuit or muffin	1

STARCH UNIT GROUP

Breads*	
†Cornbread, 2″ cube	1
English muffin	½
Hamburger bun	½
†Pancake, 5″ diameter	1
Roll, plain, 1 oz	1
Tortilla, corn or flour, 6″ diameter	1 small
Cereal	
Bran flakes	½ c
Flaked cereal	¾ c
Grape Nuts	¼ c
Shredded wheat	¾ c
Grits, cooked	½ c
Oatmeal, cooked	½ c
Wheat cereal, cooked	½ c
Wheat germ	¼ c
Crackers	
Graham, 2½″ square	2
Matzo	½
Melba toast	4 slices
Oyster	20
Rye wafers, 2″ × 3½″	3
Soda	4
Zwieback	2
Starchy Vegetables‡	
Barley	½ c
Bulgar	½ c
§‡Dried beans, cooked	½ c
§‡Dried peas, cooked	½ c
Chayote	½ c
Corn	⅓ c
Corn on cob	1 small
Jicama	½ c
Green peas	½ c
Parsnips	⅔ c
Potato, white,	small
mashed, or boiled	½ c

THE STARCH UNIT GROUP

Starchy Vegetables‡

Pumpkin	¾ c
Rice	½ c
Rutabagas	¾ c
Winter squash	½ c
Yam or sweet potato	¼ c

Flour Products

Bread crumbs, dried	3 tbsp
Bread sticks, 4″ long	2
Cornflake crumbs	3 tbsp
Cornmeal, dry	2 tbsp
Cornstarch	2 tbsp
Flour	2 tbsp
Wheat germ	¼ c
Pasta, cooked (spaghetti, noodles, or macaroni)	½ c
Popcorn, no fat added	2 c

---

* 1 bread unit = 70 calories, 15 grams carbohydrate, 2 grams protein, and 0 grams fat.
† Each unit counts as 1 bread unit *and* 1 fat unit if commercial.
‡ All vegetables are measured after they are cooked.
§ Each unit counts as 1 bread unit *and* 1 meat unit.

MEAT UNIT GROUP*

LOW FAT MEAT GROUP†

BEANS: dried beans and dried peas (counts as 1 meat unit and 1 starch unit)	½ c
BEEF: baby beef, chuck (very lean), flank and round steak, rump, and tenderloin	1 oz
COTTAGE CHEESE: lowfat	¼ c
FISH: any fresh or frozen; canned in water salmon, tuna, crab, clams, and shellfish	1 oz
LAMB: leg, rib, sirloin, loin, and shank	1 oz
PORK: leg, whole rump, or center shank	1 oz

MEET UNIT GROUP

LOW FAT MEAT GROUP†

POULTRY: chicken, turkey (skinned), cornish hen, and pheasant	1 oz
TOFU	3 oz
VEAL: leg, loin, rib, shank, or cutlets	1 oz

MEDIUM FAT MEAT GROUP‡

BEEF: ground, less than 15% fat	1 oz
CHEESE: ricotta, part skim	¼ c
mozarella, part skim	1 oz
EGG	1
LIVER	1 oz
PEANUT BUTTER, also counts as 2 additional fat units	2 tbsp
PORK: loin	1 oz

* All meat is measured after it is cooked.
† 1 meat unit = 55 calories, 0 grams carbohydrate, 7 grams protein, and 3 grams fat.
‡ 1 meat unit = 70–80 calories, 0 grams carbohydrate, 7 grams protein, and 5–6 grams fat.

HIGH FAT MEAT GROUP*

BEEF: brisket, commercial hamburger, rib roasts, and club and rib steaks†	1 oz
LAMB: breast	1 oz
PORK: spare ribs, loin (back ribs), and ground pork	1 oz
VEAL: breast	1 oz
POULTRY: duck, goose	1 oz
CHEESE: cheddar types, most cheeses	1 oz
COLD CUTS: frankfurters and bologna	1 oz

* These meat items are especially high in fat and/or salt and are not recommended for frequent use.
† 1 meat unit = 100–110 calories, 0 grams carbohydrate, 7 grams protein, and 9–10 grams fat

MILK UNIT GROUP*

‡Lowfat milk	1 c
Yogurt, lowfat, plain	1 c

MILK UNIT GROUP*

Buttermilk	1 c
†Nonfat milk	1 c
†Powdered (nonfat milk)	⅓ c
Cheese, lowfat	1½ oz

* 1 milk unit = 140 calories, 13 grams carbohydrate, 10 grams protein, and 5 grams fat.
‡ Lowfat milk has 5 grams fat per cup.
　Whole milk has 10 grams fat per cup.
　Nonfat milk has 0 grams fat per cup.
† Because of zero fat content, you may add 1 unit more of fat to your daily intake.

FAT UNIT GROUP*

Avocado, medium	⅛
Butter	1 tsp
Chocolate, unsweetened	2 tsp
Coconut, unsweetened	1 tbsp
Cream cheese	1 tbsp
Heavy cream	1 tbsp
Margarine made from safflower, corn, cottonseed, or soy oils	1 tsp
Mayonnaise	1 tsp
Oil, safflower, corn, soy, olive, or peanut	1 tsp
Nuts, no added oil	
Almonds	10 whole
Pecans	2 large whole
Walnuts	6 small
Peanuts	20 small
Peanut butter	1½ tsp
Olives, small	5
Pumpkin seeds	1 tbsp
Sour cream	2 tbsp
Sunflower seeds	2 tbsp

* 1 fat unit = 45 calories, 0 grams carbohydrate, 0 grams protein, and 5 grams fat.

VEGETABLE UNIT GROUP*

Asparagus	Escarole	Parsley
Bean sprouts	Greens:	Radishes
Beets	Beet	Rhubarb
Broccoli	Chard	Sauerkraut
Brussel sprouts	Collard	String beans
Cabbage	Dandelion	(green and wax)
Carrots	Kale	Summer squash
Cauliflower	Mustard	Tomatoes
Celery	Spinach	Tomato juice
Chicory	Turnip	Turnips
Chinese cabbage	Lettuce	Vegetable juice
Cucumbers	Mushrooms	Watercress
Eggplant	Okra	Zucchini
Endive	Onions	

* 1 vegetable unit = 1 cup which = 28 calories, 5 grams carbohydrate, 2 grams protein, and 0 grams fat.
† 1 serving is ½ cup of cooked vegetables; raw vegetables in any amount.

Free List

Raw vegetables	Limes
Beverages: coffee, tea	Gelatin, unflavored
Bouillon, broth, consommé	Vinegar
Cranberries, unsweetened	Sugarless gum
Herbs, spices	Water, plain or
Horseradish	carbonated
Lemons	

Foods to Avoid

Alcoholic beverages	"Dietetic" foods	Nondairy
Cakes	Doughnuts	creamers
Candy	Fats	Pastries
Chewing gum	Fried Foods	Pies
Chocolate (except	Fruited yogurt	Soft drinks
as listed in the	Honey	Sugar, all kinds
fat exchange list)	Jam	Sweetened
Condensed milk	Jelly	beverages

Basic Diet Plans

You will notice that the grams of carbohydrate, protein, and fat are listed for each food group for your information. However, you needn't be concerned with committing those values to memory. The approximate calorie value of the food group units is also given for your information. For example, every unit in the starch unit group is worth about 70 calories. What you must learn, however, is the portion sizes of the most common foods you eat. For example, ½ cup of rice is one unit of starch; ⅛ avocado is one unit of fat, and so forth. You will see in just a bit how the food groups fit into the basic diet plan—that is, how many units of each food group unit you can have at each meal. But first, there are two basic diet plans. There is a 1,500-calorie basic plan, for use by most people. On this plan you will lose weight in a gradual and safe manner of about 2 to 3 pounds per week. This plan is ideal for those who are combining the diet with an exercise program. Depending on your present weight, the more you weigh the faster will be your weight loss on this plan. There is another diet plan consisting of 1,200 calories for those who by necessity are less physically active, for whom the 1,500-calorie plan would cause too slow of a weight loss. It should be emphasized that ideally, a weight loss program should include not only a lowered calorie diet, and a health promoting one at that, but also physical activity. Thirty minutes of moderately intense exercise daily facilitates weight loss. Now the two Basic Diet plans:

1,500-CALORIE BASIC PLAN

Breakfast
  2 fruit units
  2 starch units
  1 fat unit
  1 milk unit

Lunch
  3 meat units
  2 starch units

1,500-CALORIE BASIC PLAN

Lunch

    1 fat unit
    vegetable units as desired
    1 milk unit
    1 fruit unit

Dinner

    3 meat units
    2 starch units
    2 fat units
    vegetable units as desired
    1 fruit unit

Note: If you wish to use nonfat milk in place of lowfat milk, you can have 1 extra fat unit for each cup of nonfat milk substituted.

1,200-CALORIE BASIC PLAN

Breakfast

    1 fruit unit
    2 starch units
    1 fat unit
    1 milk unit

Lunch

    2 meat units
    1 starch unit
    1 fat unit
    vegetable units as desired
    1 milk unit
    1 fruit unit

Dinner

    3 meat units
    1 starch unit
    1 fat unit
    vegetable units as desired
    1 fruit unit

Note: If you wish to use nonfat milk in place of lowfat milk, you can have 1 extra fat unit for each cup of nonfat milk substituted.

The basic diet plans, either 1,500 or 1,200 calories, are to be used with the six food unit groups in the following manner:
Example—1,500-calorie plan

Breakfast

   2 fruit units

1. Refer to the fruit group page. Select any 2 fruits that you wish to eat for breakfast. Consume only the quantity listed beside each fruit. For example, if you desire some bananas and orange juice, the corresponding quantity next to bananas is ½ small; next to orange juice it's ½ cup. This is the quantity of fruit allowed at breakfast.

   2 starch units

2. Refer to the starch group page. Select any 2 starches in the quantity described or select 1 starch and double the quantity. For example, if you selected oatmeal, you would be allowed 1 cup of cooked oatmeal as ½ cup is one unit, and 1 cup is 2 units. You could also have 2 slices of bread, or ½ cup of oatmeal plus 1 slice of bread.

   1 fat unit

3. Again, going to the fat group page, you may select any 1 item in the quantity listed. At breakfast, most likely you will select 1 teaspoon of butter or margarine which you could place in your oatmeal, or spread on your toast, or you may "save" the fat unit and use it at lunch or dinner as a bonus.

   1 milk unit

4. The most likely breakfast choice from this group would be 1 cup of lowfat milk. Try cooking your cereal in the milk for a richer tasting, stick-to-the-ribs breakfast. If you cannot drink milk, substitute 1½ ounces of lowfat cheese in its place. You could have the cheese for a snack later in mid-morning.

Continuing with the sample 1,500-calorie menu:

Lunch	Sample Menu
3 meat units	3 oz water-packed tuna
2 starch units	2 small sourdough rolls
1 fat unit	1 tsp oil in dressing
vegetables as desired	lettuce, tomatoes, cucumbers, or onions
1 milk unit	8 oz plain lowfat yogurt
1 fruit unit	½ c peach halves, water-packed

Dinner	
3 meat units	3 oz lean round steak
2 starch units	1 c steamed brown rice
2 fat units	1 tsp butter or margarine and 1 tsp oil for salad dressing
vegetables as desired	mixed green salad and steamed broccoli
1 fruit unit	¾ c strawberries

You can use your imagination in cooking with foods and flavorings from the Free List. The recipes and menus in the next chapter will demonstrate some ways in which you can combine foods to create gourmet specialties. You can mix foods such as starch units with meat units, or fruit units with milk units to create combination dishes. Spaghetti with meat sauce is measured out as follows if you are using the 1,500-calorie basic plan for dinner:

2 starch units = 1 c cooked spaghetti, plain

3 meat units = ¾ c lean meat sauce, as 1 oz meat is approximately ¼ c (no need to figure in the tomato sauce as these will be relatively low in calories, but do not add any extra fat to the sauce)

A fruit "milkshake" consisting of 1 cup of lowfat milk blended with 1 ripe peach would equal 1 milk unit and 1 fruit unit. By keeping track of the number of units that you've eaten from each group, you will automatically be within the 1,500-calorie range, if that is the plan you are following, or the 1,200-calorie plan. You don't actually have to count calories, just food units. However, in time, you will probably want to know the approximate calorie value of a unit of each food group as this will permit you a greater lattitude when for very special occasions you indulge a bit more.

After having studied the basic diet plans you might react by saying that they contain too much food to ever lead to weight loss. It seems that unless a diet goes down to 800 or 1,000 calories or even lower, and unless a diet is deprivational do most people think they'll lose weight. As discussed in chapter 1, there are important physiological reasons why a very low calorie diet can be counterproductive and why moderate calorie restrictions, such as on the Alive and Well Diet is advantageous. We have already discussed the psychological reasons why a higher calorie diet leads to greater success in keeping the weight off for good. Also, very low calorie diets tend to decrease your stamina and make you feel less like engaging in calorie-burning exercise. The closer your diet can be to "normal," the more apt you are to follow it for a longer time. Besides, a weight loss greater than 2 or 3 pounds per week will be mostly water and protein tissue loss. Loss of these is undesirable and provides false comfort as they are quickly put back on once the diet is discontinued.

There are a few basic tools which you will need in order to follow the diet plan you have selected.

1. Measuring cups—plastic, assorted sizes
2. Measuring spoons—teaspoon, tablespoon
3. Small ounce scale—measuring up to 1 pound is good
4. Teflon pans, large and small skillet, or nonstick pan spray

You Must Measure

It is *imperative*, and this point cannot be emphasized enough, that you measure all quantities to the amounts that are indicated on your diet. Do not "eyeball" it; not at first anyway. After several weeks of measuring, you will know what 1 cup of rice looks like, or what 3 ounces of chicken looks like. However a little bit extra at each meal could increase the daily calorie total an extra 500 calories.

Pay special attention to measuring the fat you use on the diet. Fat is the most concentrated source of calories; 1 teaspoon has about 45 calories. All foods on the diet are to be prepared without added fat, or use only the quantities of fat that your diet plan allows for that meal. For example, if you are allowed 2 fat units for dinner, you could use 1 of the fat units to sauté your fish, and use the remaining fat unit as the oil in your salad dressing. Meats such as beef, pork, chicken, and fish are to be measured after trimmed of all visible fat, boned, skinned, and cooked. Vegetable salads need not be limited to a measured quantity as these are very low in calories. However, be sure to use a low calorie dressing! The following will aid you in your measuring:

TABLE OF KITCHEN MEASURES

Fluid Measure

4 c	= 2 pt	= 1 qt	= 32 oz	
2 c	= 1 pt	= 16 oz		
1 c	= 8 oz	= 16 tbsp		
⅞ c	= 14 tbsp			
¾ c	= 12 tbsp			
⅔ c	= 10 tbsp + 2 tsp			
½ c	= 8 tbsp			
⅓ c	= 5 tbsp + 1 tsp			
¼ c	= 4 tbsp			
⅛ c	= 2 tbsp	= 1 oz		
1 tbsp	= 3 tsp	= ½ oz		

Dry Measure

1 lb	= 16 oz	= 454 g
1 oz	= approx. 30 g	
100 g	= approx. 3 oz	

Meal Frequency

The 1,500- and 1,200-calorie basic diet plans are formulated around 3 meals per day. It is important to space mealtimes about 4 or 5 hours apart. Skipping meals causes excessive hunger and what I call the bottomless pit syndrome. Even after you devour your regular lunch or dinner, you will never satisfy the "bottomless pit." There is the risk of overeating as a result. Studies have shown that when laboratory animals are divided into two groups, both being fed the same number of calories, but one group is fed once a day, and the other, several times a day, the more frequent feeders converted less of the food to fat than the once a day group. This phenomenon can conceivably happen with people. It has been my experience as a nutritionist, and the experience of several researchers, that a consistent finding among the overweight is that the overweight have fewer meals, skipping breakfast, but eating large dinners.

If you presently have no appetite in the morning it may be that that is because you overeat at dinner. Try following the diet plan at dinner carefully. More than likely, because dinner is not a heavy meal anymore, you will feel like eating at breakfast. If you are short on time in the morning to get to work, you can pack a simple breakfast and eat at the office a bit later. A small thermos of milk, a small can of juice, a plastic bag of dry cereal, or a cheese sandwich or a muffin or bread (recipes in chapter 7) make good fast breakfasts.

While there are three meals planned on both basic diet plans, snacks, consisting of food not eaten at the previous or subsequent meal may be included as desired. For example, on the 1,500-calorie plan, one of the two fruits from breakfast may be eaten between breakfast and lunch. The same applies for snacks between lunch and dinner, and between dinner and bedtime.

Milk May Not Be for Everyone

Now a word on milk. There are some individuals who cannot tolerate milk, although they can tolerate cheese, and possibly yogurt. There are some individuals who do not like the taste of milk. The first group may be lactase deficient. That is, they have a relative deficiency in the enzyme lactase which in the intestinal tract converts the milk sugar lactose into its constituent parts, the simple sugars glucose and galactose. When the enzyme that splits lactose into the two smaller sugars is not present in sufficient quantity, lactose cannot be absorbed and remains in the intestinal tract, fermenting. This leads to a feeling of nausea, bloating, cramps, and diarrhea. Because hard and semihard cheese is a cultured milk product, it does not contain lactose and therefore is not a problem for those who cannot otherwise tolerate milk. Milk products are one of the single most important sources of calcium in the diet. All too many women in America suffer from osteoporosis, a condition in which abnormal amounts of calcium are lost from bones, leading to a weaker bone structure. This bone-thinning condition ultimately affects one fourth of all women, leaving its victims with a greater susceptibility to bone fractures. One of the major contibutors to this problem is a diet lacking in calcium. Women develop osteoporosis three times as often as men. Childbearing is one reason. The growing fetus and breast-feeding take a large amount of calcium from the mother. A woman has to increase her calcium intake by almost 100 percent during pregnancy and lactation. Many women fail to do so. Another reason why women may be more deficient in calcium than men is because women may go on drastic weight reduction diets which may leave out high calcium foods. For these reasons, the following chart of milk substitutes is included for those who cannot tolerate fluid milk:

> 1 c lowfat milk is equal in calcium and calories to:
> 1½ oz lowfat cheese
> 1 c lowfat, plain yogurt
> 1 c lowfat milk is equal in calcium but not calories to:
> 1½ c cooked spinach, kale, or turnip greens
> (1½ c contains about 80 calories; lowfat milk has about 140 calories)

Use of Dietetic or Special Foods

Most of the foods which you will select on your diet will be fresh, minimally processed foods which you can purchase from your local supermarket. There are, however, a few food products which you may want to try which will either be found in the "diet" section of your supermarket, or in a large health food store. Here are a few you may want to select and where they are available:

Fructose is sugar from fruit and is sweeter than regular table sugar so you only have to use about half as much. Most supermarkets now carry it in the sugar or diet section.

Low calorie margarine is made by whipping margarine with water so that the volume is doubled. One teaspoon of low calorie margarine has half the calories of regular margarine. Therefore, you can use 2 teaspoons of the low calorie margarine in place of only 1 teaspoon of regular margarine. Found in the refrigerator section of your supermarket.

Low calorie mayonnaise is made with half the fat found in regular mayonnaise. It contains about half the calories of regular mayonnaise. Available in supermarkets.

Sugar-reduced jam or jelly contains ⅓ to ½ the calories of regular jam or jelly because the sugar content has been reduced. Found in the diet or preserves section of your market.

Egg substitutes are made from egg whites and may be used by those for whom reduction in cholesterol intake has been advised. Available in supermarkets.

Sodium-reduced soy sauce contains about half the sodium of regular soy sauce. Available in large supermarkets or health food stores.

Whole wheat and whole grain pasta products such as whole wheat noodles or corn macaroni or cracked wheat, are available in large supermarkets or health food stores. You may want to discover the robust rich flavor and nutrition of these products.

Remember that the word *dietetic* doesn't necessarily mean low calorie. A product could be salt free or specially formulated for diabetics. Sugarless candy for example, is usually made with sorbitol, a slowly metabolized sweetener that has just as many calories as sugar. Dietetic ice cream is the same story. Dietetic peanut butter may simply be salt free, but no lower in fat or calories. The pertinent information which you will need to make an informed choice is usually available on the label. Compare the calories per serving with the "non" dietetic product. On the Alive and Well Diet the use of artificial sweeteners is not encouraged. In some of the recipes which follow where sweetening is needed, fructose is used. Fructose does cost considerably more than ordinary sugar, however. The recipes use fruits as sweetening frequently.

One last word about additives, preservatives, and the use of caffeine and alcohol. The Alive and Well Diet uses unprocessed or minimally processed foods to a large extent. Fresh fruits and vegetables, frozen or plain, are preferred. Occasionally water-packed or juice-packed canned fruits are used. Fresh meats, chicken, fish, cheese, and milk are used. Breads and cereals are minimally processed, although, frequently, small quantities of preservatives or antioxidants have been added. We feel that an all things in moderation approach here is wise. Some of the additives are naturally occurring substances, and offer more benefits than harm. The same motto applies with respect to the use of coffee or tea. Occasionally the diet may be adjusted to include a glass of wine or beer. More on this in chapter 9.

7 / Menus and Recipes

In the following pages are listed 80 days of menus and 75 recipes using the lowfat, low sugar, low salt method of preparation. The menus are intended to guide you in your daily food selection. If you prefer to substitute one vegetable for another or one starch for another and so forth, you can, as long as you use the correct quantity. Each daily menu is calculated to contain 1,500 calories or less. The menus are based on the 1,500-Calorie Basic Plan shown in chapter 6, which is as follows:

1,500-CALORIE BASIC PLAN

Breakfast
>   2 fruit units
>   2 starch units
>   1 fat unit
>   1 milk unit

Lunch
>   3 meat units
>   2 starch units

1,500-CALORIE BASIC PLAN

Lunch

1 fat unit
vegetable units as desired
1 milk unit
1 fruit unit

Dinner

3 meat units
2 starch units
2 fat units
vegetable units as desired
1 fruit unit

NOTE: If you wish to use nonfat milk in place of lowfat milk, you can have 1 extra fat unit for each cup of nonfat milk substituted.

You will notice that in some of the menus that are listed, a few of the food units are arranged among the three meals slightly different than the Basic Plan. For instance, when a cereal appears at breakfast, the fat units at that meal are saved and "used" at lunch or dinner. Similarly, when an egg or another meat unit such as homemade sausage is included at breakfast, the total number of meat units for the rest of the day must be reduced. Lunch, for example, would now have 2 meat units, not 3. When you are planning for a dessert at lunch or dinner, you have to reduce that meal by the quantity of food units which are equal to the calorie value of that dessert. For 1 serving of pear cake, for example, which is 130 calories, you will have to give up about that many calories from other foods. To review the calorie values of the food units:

Food Unit	Calories
1 meat unit	55–80
1 starch unit	70
1 milk unit	140
1 fruit unit	50
1 fat unit	45
1 vegetable unit	25

Knowing that 1 starch unit is 70 calories, plus 1 fruit unit at 50 calories totals 120 calories, you could omit these 2 food units at the meal where you will have the pear cake and still be within your daily calorie allotment.

If you are following the 1,200-Calorie Basic Plan, you will have to adjust the 1,500 menus by reducing some of the food units. The 1,200-Calorie Basic Plan:

1,200-CALORIE BASIC PLAN

Breakfast
 1 fruit unit
 2 starch units
 1 fat unit
 1 milk unit

Lunch
 2 meat units
 1 starch unit
 1 fat unit
 vegetable units as desired
 1 milk unit
 1 fruit unit

Dinner
 3 meat units
 1 starch unit
 1 fat unit
 vegetable units as desired
 1 fruit unit

Note: If you wish to use nonfat milk in place of lowfat milk, you can have 1 extra fat unit for each cup of nonfat milk substituted.

Reduce the 1,500 menus by a total of:

Food Unit	Calories
1 meat unit	70
2 starch units	140
1 fat unit	45
1 fruit unit	50
Total Calories	305

This adjustment will convert the 1,500 menus into your 1,200-Calorie Basic Plan. When you are preparing recipes, you will have smaller portions for some meals as the total number of food units on the 1,200-plan are fewer than on the 1,500-plan.

I hope that you will try the taste-tested recipes, all of which were prepared on the *Alive and Well* television show. You can create your own recipes as well by using these as an example and following the guidelines in chapter 8.

Note: Asterisks in the menu section refer to recipes in this book. (See index.)

MENU 1

Calories	**BREAKFAST**
50	¼ small melon
140	⅓ c whole grain cereal, uncooked
140	1 c lowfat milk
	coffee or tea

	LUNCH
375	grilled tuna sandwich (2 slices rye bread, 2 oz tuna, 1 oz lowfat cheese, 1 tsp mayonnaise, onion, and celery)
25	assorted fresh vegetables
140	1 c lowfat milk
50	1 peach

	DINNER
340	*spinach-cheese pie
25	tomato, green pepper, onion salad
70	2 oz baby shrimp with lemon and herbs
50	¾ c strawberries
75	½ c plain yogurt with 1 tsp each of fructose and vanilla

1,480

MENU 2

Calories	**BREAKFAST**
50	½ c pineapple/grapefruit juice
150	2 slices raisin wheat toast
45	1 tsp butter or margarine
140	1 c lowfat milk
	coffee or tea

Calories	**LUNCH**
330	*tarte Niçoise
20	romaine lettuce and cucumber salad
45	1 tbsp herb dressing
140	1 c lowfat milk
50	2 apricots

Calories	**DINNER**
165	3 oz veal with tarragon
140	1 c rice pilaf
40	½ c artichoke hearts
25	1 tbsp sour cream with lemon and cayenne
15	Bibb lettuce salad
45	1 tbsp French dressing
50	1 c melon cubes

1,450

MENU 3

Calories	**BREAKFAST**
50	½ c orange juice
140	2 slices wheat toast
90	1 tbsp peanut butter
20	2 tsp sugar-reduced jam
140	1 c lowfat milk
	coffee or tea

Calories	**LUNCH**
180	3 oz meat loaf
140	2 slices whole wheat bread

25	cole slaw
45	1 tbsp vinaigrette dressing
140	1 c lowfat milk
50	1 pear

DINNER

165	*3 oz Hungarian chicken
140	1 c noodles
25	steamed broccoli and yellow squash
45	1 tsp butter or margarine
100	*tropical pineapple-meringue slices

1,495

MENU 4

Calories	BREAKFAST
50	½ c orange juice
70	1 scrambled egg
140	2 slices whole wheat toast
90	2 tsp butter or margarine
140	1 c lowfat milk
	coffee or tea

LUNCH

205	1¼ c navy bean soup
25	mixed green salad
45	1 tbsp honey-mustard dressing
70	1 small whole wheat roll
45	1 tsp butter or margarine
80	1 oz lowfat cheese
50	1 slice watermelon

DINNER

165	3 oz grilled swordfish with teriyaki sauce
140	1 c steamed brown rice
45	1 tsp butter or margarine
25	Oriental vegetables
10	sliced tomatoes
100	1 c pineapple chunks

1,495

MENU 5

Calories	**BREAKFAST**
50	1 c grapefruit juice
140	1 whole wheat English muffin
90	2 tsp butter or margarine
140	1 c lowfat milk
	coffee or tea

	LUNCH
270	baked eggplant slices with tomatoes, mushrooms and 3 oz lowfat cheese
70	1 small French roll
145	*⅔ c brown rice and raisin pudding

	DINNER
280	broiled lamb chop (4 oz boneless)
140	1 c twist noodles with chopped parsley
40	2 tsp Parmesan cheese
25	steamed broccoli with lemon
100	¼ melon with ½ c blueberries

1,490

MENU 6

Calories	**BREAKFAST**
50	½ c orange juice
140	1½ c shredded wheat
140	1 c lowfat milk
50	¾ c strawberries
	coffee or tea

	LUNCH
170	chicken salad (3 oz shredded chicken, chopped celery, parsley, and onions on lettuce bed)
45	1 tbsp honey-mustard dressing
140	2 small whole wheat rolls
45	1 tsp butter or margarine

140	1 c lowfat milk
50	2 walnut-stuffed dates

DINNER

165	*3 oz halibut marengo
70	½ c brown rice pilaf
45	1 tsp butter or margarine
15	Swiss chard with lemon juice
25	fresh vegetable salad
45	1 tbsp herb dressing
140	*orange wheat germ cake

1,475

MENU 7

Calories	BREAKFAST
50	½ c grapefruit juice
150	2 slices raisin-cinnamon toast
45	1 tsp butter or margarine
140	1 c lowfat milk
	coffee or tea

LUNCH

300	chef's salad (2 oz roast beef, 1 oz lowfat cheese, ⅓ c kidney beans, and assorted fresh vegetables on lettuce)
30	2 tbsp lemon-Dijon dressing
70	1 small sourdough roll
45	1 tsp butter or margarine
140	1 c lowfat milk
50	2 plums

DINNER

165	3 oz chicken baked with mustard and dill weed
50	⅔ c creamed rutabaga
25	steamed green beans with herbs
90	1 small corn muffin
45	1 tsp butter or margarine
100	1 c grapes

1,495

MENU 8

Calories	**BREAKFAST**
50	½ c orange juice
140	1 bagel, toasted
45	1 tbsp cream cheese
140	1 c lowfat milk
	coffee or tea

	LUNCH
330	steak sandwich (3 oz lean minute steak, 1 med French roll, and grilled onions)
25	mixed vegetable salad
35	1 tbsp green goddess dressing
140	1 c lowfat milk
50	1 apple

	DINNER
270	*cheese broccoli soup
70	small whole wheat roll
20	romaine lettuce and tomato salad
50	1 oz shrimp
45	1 tbsp herb dressing
50	¼ melon

1,460

MENU 9

Calories	**BREAKFAST**
50	1 tangerine
140	1½ c cornflakes
50	1 peach
140	1 c lowfat milk
	coffee or tea

	LUNCH
380	French bread pizza (1 long French roll, 3 oz lowfat cheese, tomato sauce, bellpepper, onions, and mushrooms)

70	marinated vegetable salad (1 tsp oil, carrots, zucchini, and cauliflower)
140	1 c lowfat milk
50	1 apple

DINNER

230	*1 c lima beans in tomato sauce
90	5-layer vegetable salad (lettuce, zucchini, red onions, cucumber, and 1 oz lowfat cheese)
45	1 tbsp honey-mustard dressing
100	1 c fresh fruit parfait

1,485

MENU 10

Calories

BREAKFAST

50	½ c orange juice
150	2 slices raisin bread
90	2 tsp butter or margarine
140	1 c lowfat milk
	coffee or tea

LUNCH

185	*3 oz *escabèche* on lettuce bed
45	1 tsp butter or margarine
140	6 small rye crackers, unsalted
140	1 c lowfat milk
50	1 peach

DINNER

385	*1 c *linguine* with eggplant and veal sauce
20	mixed green salad
45	1 tbsp vinaigrette dressing
65	1 slice California fruit torte

1,505

MENU 11

Calories	**BREAKFAST**
50	½ grapefruit
140	1½ c flaked wheat cereal
50	½ banana
140	1 c lowfat milk
	coffee or tea

	LUNCH
225	*stir-"fried" turkey (3 oz) and vegetables
45	1 tsp oil
70	½ c steamed rice
50	¼ small melon
70	2 squares whole grain graham crackers
140	1 c lowfat milk

	DINNER
290	*shepherd's beef and potato pie
20	endive and watercress salad
45	1 tbsp herb dressing
70	1 small wheat roll
45	1 tsp butter or margarine
50	10 large cherries

1,455

MENU 12

Calories	**BREAKFAST**
50	½ grapefruit
140	1½ c wheat flakes
50	½ banana
140	1 c lowfat milk
	coffee or tea

	LUNCH
230	open-faced cheese sandwich (1 slice pumpernickel bread, and 2 oz lowfat cheese)

140	marinated bean salad (½ c kidney beans, celery, and onions on lettuce)
45	1 tbsp herb dressing
140	1 c lowfat milk
50	1 peach

DINNER

195	*cioppino*
70	½ c steamed rice
70	1 small sourdough roll
25	"sautéed" zucchini
90	2 tsp butter or margarine
50	apple and orange salad (½ apple and ½ orange)

1,485

MENU 13

Calories

BREAKFAST

50	½ c orange juice
140	1½ c shredded wheat
140	1 c lowfat milk
50	½ banana
	coffee or tea

LUNCH

330	turkey (2 oz) and cheese (1 oz) on whole wheat bun
20	lettuce, tomatoes, and sprouts
45	1 tbsp mayonnaise
140	1 c lowfat milk
50	2 plums

DINNER

305	*New England clam chowder
20	endive and watercress salad
45	1 tbsp French dressing
70	1 sourdough roll
75	⅔ c apples and raisins in orange juice

1,480

MENU 14

Calories	**BREAKFAST**
50	½ c orange juice
210	2 slices French toast (2 slices whole wheat bread and 1 egg)
60	1 tbsp butter or margarine
20	2 tsp sugar-reduced syrup
140	1 c lowfat milk
	coffee or tea

Calories	**LUNCH**
125	crab salad (3 oz crab, lettuce, and tomatoes)
15	1 tbsp lemon-Dijon dressing
140	2 small rolls
45	1 tsp butter or margarine
140	1 c lowfat milk
50	1 slice watermelon

Calories	**DINNER**
170	3 oz sliced leg of lamb
140	1 c onioned Bulgar pilaf
60	½ c steamed peas with mushrooms
20	mixed vegetable salad
45	1 tbsp herb dressing
50	1 baked apple

1,480

MENU 15

Calories	**BREAKFAST**
50	1 orange, sectioned
140	½ c Grape Nuts
50	½ banana
140	1 c lowfat milk
	coffee or tea

Calories	**LUNCH**
330	cheeseburger on whole wheat bun (2 oz lean beef pattie and 1 oz lowfat cheese)

10	sliced tomato, lettuce, and onions
75	⅔ c apple, carrot, and raisin salad
20	1 tbsp sour cream dressing
140	1 c lowfat milk

DINNER

230	*red snapper San Diego
140	2 small oven-baked potatoes
45	1 tsp butter or margarine
20	steamed green beans and cauliflower
15	romaine lettuce
20	1 tbsp cucumber dressing
50	½ c fresh fruit compote

1,475

MENU 16

Calories	**BREAKFAST**
50	½ c orange juice
140	⅓ c whole wheat cereal, uncooked
140	1 c lowfat milk
50	2 tbsp raisins
	coffee or tea

LUNCH

335	2 chicken tostadas (2 corn tortillas, 2 oz shredded chicken, 1 oz lowfat cheese, lettuce, tomato, onions, and ¼ avocado)
20	1 tbsp sour cream
140	1 c lowfat milk
50	½ papaya

DINNER

240	*beef- and rice-stuffed tomatoes
140	Mediterranean salad (lettuce, cucumber, onions, green pepper, 6 olives, and 1 oz crumbled cheese)
70	1 tbsp vinaigrette dressing
50	1 small roll
45	½ c peach slices

1,470

MENU 17

Calories	BREAKFAST
50	½ c grapefruit juice
140	1½ c shredded wheat
50	½ banana
140	1 c lowfat milk
	coffee or tea

Calories	LUNCH
315	3 oz sliced turkey on 2 slices rye with sliced tomatoes and sprouts
25	1 tsp mayonnaise
45	assorted fresh vegetables
190	fruit shake (1 c lowfat milk blended with ½ c raspberries or other fruit

Calories	DINNER
165	3 oz broiled salmon with lemon-herb sauce
230	oven-fried potatoes (2 small potatoes and 2 tsp butter)
25	steamed greens (collard, turnip, or mustard)
120	*citron Alaska

1,495

MENU 18

Calories	BREAKFAST
50	½ c orange/pineapple juice
70	1 poached egg
140	2 slices wheat toast
45	1 tsp butter or margarine
140	1 c lowfat milk
	coffee or tea

Calories	LUNCH
260	French dip beef sandwich (1 French roll and 2 oz roast beef)
25	shredded celery root salad

45	1 tsp mayonnaise
140	1 c lowfat milk
50	½ c grapes

DINNER

165	barbequed chicken (3 oz)
90	1 corn on the cob
45	1 tsp butter or margarine
70	1 small wheat roll
20	fresh vegetable salad
15	1 tbsp lemon-Dijon dressing
110	*fresh strawberry pie

1,480

MENU 19

Calories **BREAKFAST**

50	½ c orange/pineapple juice
140	1½ c cornflakes
50	½ banana
140	1 c lowfat milk
	coffee or tea

LUNCH

315	turkey (3 oz) on whole grain bread with lettuce, tomatoes, and sprouts
45	1 tsp mayonnaise
25	fresh vegetable plate
140	1 c lowfat milk
50	1 nectarine

DINNER

340	*Sicilian veal with pasta
20	"sautéed" zucchini
20	marinated vegetables on lettuce
45	1 tbsp herb dressing
120	berry parfait (¾ c berries and ½ c plain yogurt)

1,500

MENU 20

Calories	**BREAKFAST**
50	½ c grapefruit sections
140	2 whole grain pancakes
30	1 tbsp sugar-reduced syrup
45	1 tsp butter or margarine
70	*1 homemade pork sausage patty
140	1 c lowfat milk
	coffee or tea

Calories	**LUNCH**
260	2 open-faced grilled cheese and mushroom sandwiches (2 oz lowfat cheese, 2 slices wheat bread, and mushrooms)
20	fresh spinach salad
45	1 tbsp honey-mustard dressing
140	1 c lowfat milk
50	½ c fruited gelatin dessert (unsweetened fruit juice and fruit in gelatin)

Calories	**DINNER**
350	*chicken *couscous*
25	cucumber and parsley salad
45	1 tbsp vinaigrette dressing
50	1 nectarine

1,460

MENU 21

Calories	**BREAKFAST**
50	½ c orange juice
50	¾ c strawberries
140	1½ c cornflakes
140	1 c lowfat milk
	coffee or tea

Calories	**LUNCH**
190	Chinese chicken salad (3 oz chicken, *bokchoy*, Chinese cabbage, and bean sprouts)

45	2 tsp slivered almonds
45	1 tbsp ginger dressing
140	2 small rolls
140	1 c lowfat milk
50	½ c grapes

DINNER

225	*layered cod and spinach loaf
70	1 small parsley boiled potato
45	1 tsp butter or margarine
25	marinated beet salad
45	1 tbsp vinaigrette dressing
100	strawberry meringue

1,500

MENU 22

Calories	**BREAKFAST**
50	¼ small cantaloupe
80	¼ c ricotta cheese, part skim
140	2 slices whole wheat toast
45	1 tsp butter or margarine
140	1 c lowfat milk
	coffee or tea

LUNCH

205	curried chicken salad (3 oz chicken, 2 tbsp plain yogurt, celery, and curry on lettuce)
140	2 small whole wheat rolls
45	1 tsp butter or margarine
140	1 c lowfat milk
50	½ c pineapple chunks

DINNER

250	*sukiyaki
140	1 c steamed rice
50	½ c citrus fruit sections

1,475

MENU 23

Calories	**BREAKFAST**
50	½ c orange juice
210	*2 slices peanut butter bread
140	1 c lowfat milk
	coffee or tea

	LUNCH
380	bean and cheese burrito (1 large flour tortilla, ⅓ c pinto beans, 1½ oz lowfat cheese, and ⅛ avocado)
20	lettuce and tomato salad
10	1 tbsp cucumber dressing
140	1 c lowfat milk
50	¼ melon

	DINNER
210	broiled lamb chop (3 oz boneless)
140	1 c brown rice pilaf
25	summer squash medley
20	mixed green salad
45	1 tbsp honey-mustard dressing
50	½ c applesauce

1,490

MENU 24

Calories	**BREAKFAST**
50	½ c grapefruit juice
140	2 slices whole wheat toast
150	cheese omelet (1 egg and 1 oz lowfat cheese)
45	1 tsp butter or margarine
140	1 c lowfat milk
	coffee or tea

	LUNCH
120	*1¼ c lentil spinach soup
70	1 small wheat roll
45	1 tsp butter or margarine

140	1 c lowfat milk
50	1 peach

DINNER

240	3 oz boneless pork chops with ½ c sliced apples
70	½ c noodles
70	½ c steamed acorn squash
45	1 tsp butter or margarine
25	mixed vegetable salad
45	1 tbsp ginger dressing
50	1 plum

1,495

MENU 25

Calories	BREAKFAST
50	½ c orange juice
140	2 whole grain rolls
90	2 tsp butter or margarine
20	2 tsp sugar-reduced jam
140	1 c lowfat milk
	coffee or tea

LUNCH

305	tuna salad in pita bread (3 oz tuna, chopped parsley, celery, and onions)
45	1 tsp mayonnaise
20	assorted fresh vegetables
140	1 c lowfat milk
50	2 small apricots

DINNER

220	*veal Parmesan (3 oz)
140	1 c brown rice
25	steamed broccoli with lemon
20	mixed vegetable salad
45	1 tbsp herb dressing
50	½ c fresh fruit cup

1,500

MENU 26

Calories	
	BREAKFAST
140	1 c lowfat milk
50	1 peach
50	1 slice melon
140	4 whole grain graham cracker squares
	LUNCH
235	3 oz turkey on 2 slices rye bread
90	¼ avocado
5	sliced tomatoes, sprouts, and lettuce
140	1 c lowfat milk
120	*apple oatmeal cookies
	DINNER
340	*clam risotto
25	steamed green beans with mushrooms
20	mixed vegetable salad
45	1 tbsp herb dressing
70	½ c raspberry gele with "sour cream" icing
1,470	

MENU 27

Calories	
	BREAKFAST
50	½ c grapefruit juice
140	1 whole grain English muffin
80	¼ c ricotta cheese, part skim
20	2 tsp sugar-reduced jam
140	1 c lowfat milk
	coffee or tea
	LUNCH
70	egg salad (1 egg, chopped celery, onions, bellpepper, and parsley)
45	1 tsp mayonnaise
140	2 slices whole grain bread

20	spinach salad
45	1 tbsp honey-mustard dressing
140	1 c lowfat milk
50	¾ c strawberries

DINNER

240	beef rump roast (4 oz)
70	1 small baked potato
45	2 tbsp sour cream
25	steamed crookneck squash
150	chocolate cheese cake

1,490

MENU 28

Calories

BREAKFAST

50	½ c pineapple/grapefruit juice
140	⅓ c oatmeal, uncooked
140	1 c lowfat milk
	coffee or tea

LUNCH

165	*3 oz seviche
140	1 med French roll
45	1 tsp butter or margarine
25	artichoke and tomato salad
45	1 tbsp vinaigrette dressing
140	1 c lowfat milk
50	½ banana

DINNER

240	*beef stroganoff
140	1 c noodles
25	½ c whole baby carrots
25	romaine lettuce salad
45	1 tbsp honey-mustard dressing
50	½ c kiwi fruit and grapefruit sections

1,465

MENU 29

Calories	**BREAKFAST**
50	½ c orange juice
140	½ Grape Nuts
25	1 tbsp raisins
140	1 c lowfat milk

	LUNCH
45	1 c hot V-8 juice
300	grilled cheese sandwich (2 oz cheese and 2 slices whole grain bread)
45	1 tsp butter or margarine
25	cabbage and vegetable slaw
45	1 tbsp vinaigrette dressing
140	1 c lowfat milk
50	¼ small melon

	DINNER
255	*chicken Florentine
140	2 small potatoes, sautéed
45	1 tsp butter or margarine
15	sliced tomatoes
50	3 pineapple rings

1,510

MENU 30

Calories	**BREAKFAST**
50	1 tangerine
140	2 slices whole grain toast
90	2 tsp butter or margarine
20	2 tsp sugar-reduced jam
140	1 c lowfat milk
	coffee or tea

	LUNCH
390	*pasta salad on lettuce leaf

140	1 c lowfat milk
50	¼ small melon

DINNER

255	*3 oz stir-"fried" pork with vegetables
140	1 c steamed brown rice
70	fresh fruit parfait (½ c fruit and 2 tbsp plain yogurt)

1,485

MENU 31

Calories

BREAKFAST

50	½ c orange juice
140	1 toasted bagel
45	1 tbsp cream cheese
140	1 c lowfat milk
	coffee or tea

LUNCH

30	1 c garden vegetable soup
280	chef's salad (2 oz roast beef, 1 oz lowfat cheese, ¼ c garbanzo beans, assorted fresh vegetables and lettuce)
30	2 tbsp lemon-Dijon dressing
70	1 small whole wheat roll
45	1 tsp butter or margarine
140	1 c lowfat milk
50	1 pear

DINNER

340	*Mexican chicken and cheese casserole
20	steamed zucchini
15	mixed green salad
45	1 tbsp herb dressing
50	½ mango

1,490

MENU 32

Calories	BREAKFAST
50	½ c orange juice
140	⅓ c whole wheat cereal, uncooked
140	1 c lowfat milk
	coffee or tea

	LUNCH
340	bean and cheese burrito (1 flour tortilla, ⅓ c beans, and 1½ oz cheese)
45	1 tsp butter or margarine
20	lettuce and tomato salad
45	1 tbsp herb dressing
140	1 c lowfat milk
50	2 apricots

	DINNER
220	*salmon with wine and vegetable sauce
140	2 small parsley boiled potatoes
45	1 tsp butter or margarine
20	steamed Brussels sprouts with lemon
100	fresh fruit parfait (½ banana and 1 orange)

1,495

MENU 33

Calories	BREAKFAST
50	½ c orange juice
140	1½ c shredded wheat
50	½ banana
140	1 c lowfat milk
	coffee or tea

	LUNCH
165	3 oz cold baked chicken
140	2 whole wheat rolls
45	1 tsp butter or margarine

25	*broccoli combination salad
140	1 c lowfat milk
50	1 peach

DINNER

165	3 oz lean pot roast
140	1 c mashed potatoes
45	1 tsp butter or margarine
35	stewed carrots, celery, and onions
25	endive and watercress salad
45	1 tbsp honey-mustard dressing
50	2 red plums

1,450

MENU 34

Calories	BREAKFAST
50	½ grapefruit
140	⅓ c oatmeal, uncooked
50	2 tbsp raisins
140	1 c lowfat milk
	coffee or tea

LUNCH

260	tuna antipasto salad (salad greens with 1 oz lowfat cheese, 2 oz tuna, ¼ c navy beans, tomatoes, and cucumbers)
45	6 olives
45	1 tbsp herb dressing
70	4 melba toast
140	1 c lowfat milk
50	½ c applesauce

DINNER

210	3 oz broiled steak with grilled onions
140	2 slices toasted garlic bread
45	1 tsp butter or margarine
25	string beans in tomato sauce
60	1 pear in 1 tbsp sherry

1,490

MENU 35

Calories	**BREAKFAST**
50	1 tangerine
70	1 poached egg
140	2 slices whole wheat toast
45	1 tsp butter or margarine
140	1 c lowfat milk
	coffee or tea

	LUNCH
170	½ c herbed ricotta cheese, part skim
140	8 whole wheat melba toast
25	fresh vegetable salad (zucchini, cauliflower, carrots, and radishes)
45	1 tbsp honey-mustard dressing
140	1 c lowfat milk
50	1 persimmon

	DINNER
165	*seafood kabobs
140	1 c brown rice pilaf
60	*stuffed eggplant
15	romaine lettuce salad
15	1 tbsp lemon-Dijon dressing
50	½ c pineapple chunks

1,460

MENU 36

Calories	**BREAKFAST**
50	½ c orange juice
140	⅓ c wheat cereal, uncooked
140	1 c lowfat milk
50	½ banana
	coffee or tea

LUNCH

180	3 oz sliced beef
140	2 slices whole grain bread
25	marinated vegetable salad
45	1 tbsp vinaigrette dressing
140	1 c lowfat milk
50	2 apricots

DINNER

165	½ roasted Cornish hen
70	½ c baked acorn squash with ginger
70	½ c peas and mushrooms
45	1 tsp butter or margarine
25	spinach salad
45	1 tbsp honey-mustard dressing
120	*1 slice "light" banana cream pie

1,500

MENU 37

Calories

BREAKFAST

50	½ grapefruit
150	2 slices whole wheat raisin toast
45	1 tsp butter or margarine
140	1 c lowfat milk
	coffee or tea

LUNCH

375	grilled tuna sandwich (2 slices rye bread, 2 oz tuna, 1 tsp mayonnaise, 1 oz lowfat cheese, and onions)
20	cucumber and tomato salad
45	1 tbsp vinaigrette dressing
140	1 c lowfat milk
50	1 apple

DINNER

180	3 oz turkey meatloaf
140	1 large baked potato

20	1 tbsp sour cream
20	steamed Swiss chard
20	marinated salad (zucchini, carrots, onions, celery, and bellpepper)
45	1 tbsp herb dressing
50	½ c fruit cocktail

1,490

MENU 38

Calories

BREAKFAST

50	½ cup orange juice
140	1½ cups corn flakes
50	½ cup sliced peaches
140	1 cup low fat milk
	coffee or tea

LUNCH

175	1¼ cup split pea soup
230	toasted cheese sandwich (1 slice wheat bread, 2 ounces low fat cheese)
15	assorted raw vegetables
140	low fat milk
150	1 pear

DINNER

335	*baked shrimp stuffed pasta shells
20	steamed green beans with lemon and herbs
20	mixed vegetable salad
44	tbsp herb dressing
20	⅔ berries

1,460

MENU 39

Calories

BREAKFAST

50	½ grapefruit
140	1 whole wheat bagel

45	1 tbsp cream cheese
140	1 c lowfat milk
	coffee or tea

LUNCH

210	Joe's special (3 oz leanest sautéed ground beef with spinach and onions)
140	1 med sourdough roll, toasted
45	1 tsp butter or margarine
140	1 c lowfat milk
100	1 small banana

DINNER

370	*vegetable cassoulet
20	green salad
45	1 tsp Italian dressing
50	1 nectarine

1,495

MENU 40

Calories	BREAKFAST
50	½ c orange juice
140	1½ c wheat flakes
50	2 tbsp raisins
140	1 c lowfat milk
	coffee or tea

LUNCH

165	3 oz broiled fish fillet with herbs
140	1 c brown rice
45	1 tsp butter or margarine
20	coleslaw
45	1 tsp oil
140	1 c lowfat milk
50	1 nectarine

DINNER

195	*3 oz savory beef roll
140	1 c oven-baked potatoes

45	1 tsp butter or margarine
25	steamed zucchini, cauliflower, or carrots
15	Bibb lettuce salad
45	1 tbsp ginger dressing
50	½ c blueberries

1,500

MENU 41

Calories

BREAKFAST

50	½ grapefruit
140	⅓ c whole grain cereal, uncooked
140	1 c lowfat milk
50	2 tbsp raisins
	coffee or tea

LUNCH

165	turkey salad sandwich (3 oz turkey, 1 tbsp yogurt, green onions, and celery)
90	2 tsp mayonnaise
140	2 slices whole wheat bread
15	lettuce, tomatoes, and sprouts
140	1 c lowfat milk
50	1 nectarine

DINNER

170	*6 oysters Bienville style
140	1 c brown rice pilaf
45	1 tsp butter or margarine
20	steamed spinach with lemon
15	red radish and cucumber salad
45	1 tbsp vinaigrette dressing
50	½ c plum, peach and pear compote

1,465

MENU 42

Calories

BREAKFAST

| 50 | 1 tangerine |
| 160 | 2 buckwheat waffles (5" square) |

45	1 tsp butter or margarine
50	½ c applesauce
140	1 c lowfat milk
	coffee or tea

LUNCH

140	⅔ c black-eyed peas
70	½ c brown rice
135	cornbread, 2" x 2" x 1"
20	collard greens with lemon
45	1 tsp butter or margarine
140	1 c lowfat milk
50	2 apricots

DINNER

270	chicken soup (2 oz chicken, 1 c cooked pasta, and vegetables)
20	romaine lettuce and green onion salad
45	1 tbsp French dressing
50	½ c blackberries
40	¼ c plain lowfat yogurt, and ½ tsp fructose, and vanilla

1,500

MENU 43

Calories	**BREAKFAST**
50	½ c orange juice
140	1½ c shredded wheat
50	¾ c strawberries
140	1 c lowfat milk
	coffee or tea

LUNCH

200	cheeseburger (2 oz lean beef patty and 1 oz lowfat cheese)
140	1 whole grain bun
10	sliced tomato and onions
	mustard and catsup

20	carrot and cabbage slaw
10	1 tbsp buttermilk dressing
140	1 c lowfat milk
50	½ c pineapple

DINNER

165	3 oz broiled halibut steak
140	1 baked potato with chives
45	2 tbsp sour cream
20	steamed asparagus with lemon
15	endive and mushroom salad
45	1 tbsp ginger dressing
110	*⅔ c raspberry sherbet

1,490

MENU 44

Calories

BREAKFAST

50	½ c grapefruit juice
70	½ c grits
70	1 egg, scrambled
70	1 slice whole wheat toast
45	1 tsp butter or margarine
140	1 c lowfat milk
	coffee or tea

LUNCH

165	crab salad (3 oz crab, and assorted green lettuce, cucumbers, and tomatoes)
15	2 tbsp cucumber dressing
140	2 small sourdough rolls
45	1 tsp butter or margarine
50	1 apple

SNACK

130	½ c lowfat cottage cheese with herbs assorted fresh vegetables

DINNER

240	3 oz braised lamb chop with green beans and tomato sauce
70	½ c brown rice pilaf
20	shredded celery root salad
35	1 tbsp green goddess dressing
145	*glazed peach pie

1,500

MENU 45

Calories **BREAKFAST**

50	½ c orange/grapefruit juice
140	⅓ c oatmeal, uncooked
140	1 c lowfat milk
50	2 dates, chopped
	coffee or tea

LUNCH

180	hot chicken and cheese open-faced sandwich (2 oz chicken slices, 1 oz lowfat cheese, shredded, and tomato slices)
140	2 slices rye bread
45	⅛ avocado
20	zucchini, celery, bellpepper salad
45	1 tbsp herb dressing
140	1 c lowfat milk
50	½ c grapes

DINNER

275	*pork and bean bake
70	1 small wheat roll
45	1 tsp butter or margarine
20	mixed green salad
10	1 tbsp buttermilk dressing
50	1 pear

1,470

MENU 46

Calories	**BREAKFAST**
50	½ c orange juice
140	1 whole wheat English muffin
80	¼ c ricotta cheese, part skim
20	2 tsp sugar-reduced jam
140	1 c lowfat milk
	coffee or tea

	LUNCH
150	1¼ c potato and leek soup
230	open-faced veal loaf sandwich (3 oz veal loaf and 1 slice whole grain bread)
20	marinated green bean salad
45	1 tbsp vinaigrette dressing
50	1 apple
80	1 oz lowfat cheese

	DINNER
190	3 oz baked sea bass with tomatoes and onions
70	½ c bulgar pilaf
15	steamed zucchini with lemon
15	mixed vegetable salad
45	1 tbsp honey-mustard dressing
130	*pear cake

1,470

MENU 47

Calories	**BREAKFAST**
50	1 orange
140	⅓ c rolled oats, uncooked
140	1 c lowfat milk
50	½ banana
	coffee or tea

	LUNCH
125	shrimp and spinach salad (3 oz shrimp)
45	1 tbsp Italian dressing

140	2 small sourdough rolls
90	2 tsp butter or margarine
140	1 c lowfat milk
100	1 c grapes

DINNER

325	*cornbread-topped beef and chile casserole
15	steamed button squash
20	mixed green salad
45	1 tbsp honey-mustard dressing
50	1 tangerine

1,475

MENU 48

Calories   **BREAKFAST**

50	½ c orange/pineapple juice
140	1½ c cornflakes
50	½ c sliced peaches
140	1 c lowfat milk
	coffee or tea

LUNCH

330	beef in pita bread (3 oz sliced beef, 1 med pita bread, tomatoes, lettuce, and onions)
50	½ c yogurt with shredded cucumber
75	⅔ c shredded carrot-apple raisin salad
45	1 tsp mayonnaise
140	1 c lowfat milk

DINNER

180	*Cantonese chicken
140	1 c steamed brown rice
25	steamed snow peas
15	tomato and cucumber salad
45	1 tbsp vinaigrette dressing
65	¾ c kiwi and grapefruit sections

1,490

MENU 49

Calories	**BREAKFAST**
50	½ grapefruit
80	1 Spanish omelet
140	2 slices whole wheat toast
90	2 tsp butter or margarine
140	1 c lowfat milk
	coffee or tea

Calories	**LUNCH**
165	3 oz poached white fish with parsley sauce (parsley, onion, celery, yogurt, and pepper)
140	2 small sourdough rolls
25	marinated beet salad
45	1 tbsp herb dressing
140	1 c lowfat milk
50	2 apricots

Calories	**DINNER**
180	3 oz grilled pork chop
70	½ c noodles
45	1 tsp butter or margarine
70	½ c winter squash with ginger
15	steamed dandelion greens with lemon
50	½ c fruit cup
1,495	

MENU 50

Calories	**BREAKFAST**
50	1 tangerine
140	2 slices whole wheat toast
90	1 tbsp peanut butter
20	2 tsp sugar-reduced jam
140	1 c lowfat milk
	coffee or tea

LUNCH

210	3 oz barbecued beef
140	1 whole wheat bun
20	mixed vegetable salad
35	1 tbsp buttermilk dressing
140	1 c lowfat milk
50	½ mango

PARTY DINNER

160	*vegetable studel
70	1 oz cocktail meatballs
25	assorted fresh vegetables with light dips
70	3 rye crackers
90	4 oz white wine
60	1 c melon and strawberries

1,510

MENU 51

Calories

BREAKFAST

50	1 tangerine
140	⅓ c oatmeal, uncooked
140	1 c lowfat milk
50	2 tbsp raisins
	coffee or tea

LUNCH

145	tomato, mushroom, cheese omelet
	(1 egg and ¼ c lowfat cottage cheese)
140	2 small wheat rolls
90	2 tsp butter or margarine
20	romaine lettuce salad
45	1 tbsp vinaigrette dressing
140	1 c lowfat milk
50	1 peach

DINNER

215	*albondigas soup (meatball soup)
140	3 corn tortillas

20	coleslaw
25	1 tbsp sour cream dressing
50	½ mango with lime wedge
1,460	

MENU 52

Calories	BREAKFAST
50	½ c orange/pineapple juice
70	1 poached egg
140	2 slices wheat toast
45	1 tsp butter or margarine
140	1 c lowfat milk
	coffee or tea

	LUNCH
300	macaroni and cheese (1 c macaroni and 2 oz lowfat cheese)
25	mixed vegetable salad
45	1 tbsp Italian dressing
140	1 c lowfat milk
50	⅔ c berries

	DINNER
210	*3 oz chicken livers paysanne
140	1 c steamed rice
25	endive and shredded carrot salad
45	1 tbsp honey-mustard dressing
50	½ c pineapple-banana parfait
1,475	

MENU 53

Calories	BREAKFAST
50	½ c orange juice
140	1 whole wheat bagel
80	¼ c ricotta cheese, part skim
140	1 c lowfat milk
	coffee or tea

LUNCH

140	salmon salad (2 oz salmon and assorted vegetables)
30	2 tbsp lemon-Dijon dressing
140	1 med French roll
45	1 tsp butter or margarine
140	1 c lowfat milk
50	½ c pineapple chunks

DINNER

200	3 oz brandy-marinated steak
70	½ c oven-browned potatoes
45	1 tsp butter or margarine
45	steamed broccoli with lowfat cheese sauce
20	cucumber and watercress salad
45	1 tbsp herb dressing
85	*striped fruit gel

1,465

MENU 54

Calories
BREAKFAST

50	½ grapefruit
300	toasted cheese sandwich (2 slices rye bread, 2 oz lowfat cheese, and alfalfa sprouts) coffee or tea

LUNCH

120	*1¼ c lentil-spinach soup
180	2 corn muffins
45	1 tsp butter or margarine
140	1 c lowfat milk
50	1 pear

DINNER

240	3 oz liver sautéed with onions
70	½ small acorn stuffed squash
70	½ c peas
45	1 tsp butter or margarine
20	mixed green salad

35	1 tbsp green goddess dressing
100	1 c fresh fruit

1,465

MENU 55

Calories **BREAKFAST**
50	½ c orange juice
140	1½ c cornflakes
50	½ banana
140	1 c lowfat milk
	coffee or tea

LUNCH
165	hot turkey sandwich (3 oz sliced turkey *au jus*)
140	2 slices wheat toast
25	steamed Brussels sprouts
45	1 tsp butter or margarine
140	1 c lowfat milk
50	½ c grapes

DINNER
200	*executive crab casserole
140	1 c brown rice pilaf
25	mixed green salad
45	1 tbsp French dressing
100	1 c apricot and orange sections

1,455

MENU 56

Calories **BREAKFAST**
50	1 tangelo
140	1 whole wheat English Muffin
90	2 tsp butter or margarine
20	2 tsp sugar-reduced jam
140	1 c lowfat milk
	coffee or tea

LUNCH

180	3 oz veal patty
140	1 wheat pita bread
20	cucumber, tomato, bellpepper salad
45	1 tbsp vinaigrette dressing
140	1 c lowfat milk
50	⅓ papaya

DINNER

180	*3 oz Rosemary chicken
70	½ c mashed potatoes
25	½ c steamed baby carrots
70	1 small wheat roll
45	1 tsp butter or margarine
15	red leaf lettuce salad
10	1 tbsp buttermilk dressing
50	½ c berries

1,480

MENU 57

Calories	BREAKFAST
50	½ grapefruit
140	2 slices whole wheat toast
90	2 tsp butter or margarine
20	1 c lowfat milk
	coffee or tea

LUNCH

320	steak sandwich (1 med French roll and 3 oz sliced steak *au jus*)
25	mixed green salad
35	1 tbsp green goddess dressing
140	1 c lowfat milk
50	1 pear

DINNER

335	*layered cheese enchilada
20	steamed zucchini
20	coleslaw

45	1 tbsp vinaigrette dressing
50	⅓ papaya with lime juice

1,480

MENU 58

Calories

BREAKFAST
50	½ c orange juice
140	⅓ c wheat cereal, uncooked
140	1 c lowfat milk
50	2 dates
	coffee or tea

LUNCH
345	potato salad stuffed turkey slices (3 oz turkey, 1 c potato salad made with 1 tsp mayonnaise, and 1 tbsp lowfat yogurt)
25	marinated vegetable salad
45	1 tbsp vinaigrette dressing
140	1 c lowfat milk
50	1 apple

DINNER
230	*stefado (Greek beef and onion stew)
140	1 c rice pilaf
45	1 tsp butter or margarine
20	mixed green salad
5	1 tbsp cucumber dressing
50	¼ melon

1,475

MENU 59

Calories

BREAKFAST
50	½ c orange juice
140	1½ c shredded wheat
140	1 c lowfat milk
50	½ banana
	coffee or tea

LUNCH

185	tuna salad (3 oz tuna and assorted vegetables)
30	2 tbsp lemon-Dijon dressing
140	2 small wheat rolls
45	1 tsp butter or margarine
140	1 c lowfat milk
50	½ c grapes

DINNER

310	chili beans (½ c cooked beans and 2 oz ground beef)
70	1 small sourdough roll
20	fresh spinach salad
45	1 tbsp French dressing
65	½ c fresh fruit with 2 tbsp yogurt

1,480

MENU 60

Calories	**BREAKFAST**
50	½ grapefruit
70	1 egg omelet
70	1 small potato, hashed
90	2 tsp butter or margarine
70	1 slice wheat toast
70	½ c lowfat milk
	coffee or tea

LUNCH

280	macaroni and cheese (1 c macaroni and 2 oz lowfat cheese)
25	broiled tomato halves
100	1 c apple, raisin, pineapple salad
15	2 tbsp yogurt dressing
140	1 c lowfat milk

DINNER

150	3 oz broiled scallops
140	1 c rice pilaf
45	1 tsp butter or margarine

20	steamed green beans
15	cabbage and carrot slaw
10	1 tbsp buttermilk dressing
90	*"light" chocolate mousse

1,450

MENU 61

Calories   **BREAKFAST**

50	½ c orange juice
140	⅓ c oatmeal, uncooked
50	½ c sliced baked apples
140	1 c lowfat milk
	coffee or tea

LUNCH

350	steak and noodle twist salad (3 oz sliced flank steak, 1 c noodle twists, red bellpepper, celery, and green onions on romaine lettuce)
70	2 tbsp green goddess dressing
140	1 c lowfat milk
50	1 pear

DINNER

5	clear chicken broth and lemon soup
310	*2 chicken and shrimp egg rolls
25	stir-fried Oriental vegetables
70	½ c "fried" rice
50	½ c tangerine slices

1,450

MENU 62

Calories   **BREAKFAST**

50	½ grapefruit
140	1 whole wheat English muffin
90	1 tbsp peanut butter

50	½ banana, sliced
140	1 c lowfat milk
	coffee or tea

LUNCH

120	1¼ c minestrone soup
140	open-faced egg salad sandwich (1 slice rye bread, 1 egg with condiments, and
45	1 tsp mayonnaise)
10	sliced tomatoes and cucumbers
10	1 tbsp buttermilk dressing
140	1 c lowfat milk
50	2 apricots

DINNER

170	*3 oz Polynesian fish fillet
70	½ c rice pilaf
70	½ c winter squash with ginger
45	1 tsp butter or margarine
25	vegetable slaw (cabbage, carrots, onion, and apples)
45	1 tbsp vinaigrette dressing
50	½ mango

1,460

MENU 63

Calories	BREAKFAST
50	1 tangelo
245	*2 oatmeal muffins
140	1 c lowfat milk
	coffee or tea

LUNCH

200	2 oz roast beef and 1 oz cheese
140	2 slices wheat bread
10	lettuce and tomatoes
20	marinated vegetable salad
45	1 tbsp vinaigrette dressing
140	1 c lowfat milk
50	½ c pineapple

DINNER

190	*turkey kabobs
185	2 potato pancakes
15	steamed broccoli with lemon
15	mixed green salad
3	1 tbsp Lo-Cal tomato dressing
50	½ c fresh fruit

1,498

MENU 64

Calories	BREAKFAST
50	½ c orange juice
140	1½ c cornflakes
50	½ banana
140	1 c lowfat milk
	coffee or tea

LUNCH

350	*magic crust shrimp pie
25	mixed vegetable salad
10	1 tbsp cucumber dressing
140	1 c lowfat milk
50	2 apricots

DINNER

180	3 oz chicken in teriyaki sauce
140	1 c seasoned steamed rice
20	Oriental vegetables
90	1 tsp each butter and oil
20	Bibb lettuce and mushroom salad
45	1 tbsp ginger dressing
50	2 plums

1,500

MENU 65

Calories	BREAKFAST
50	½ c orange/grapefruit juice
140	1 whole wheat bagel

45	1 tbsp cream cheese
140	1 c lowfat milk
	coffee or tea

LUNCH

385	turkey, cheese, avocado, tomato sandwich (2 oz turkey, 1 oz lowfat cheese, ⅛ avocado, and 2 slices whole grain bread)
10	lettuce wedge
140	1 c lowfat milk
100	1 small banana

DINNER

180	3 oz baked fish with tomatoes, bellpeppers, onions, and celery
20	steamed greens with lemon
25	marinated beet salad
45	1 tbsp vinaigrette dressing
70	1 small roll
135	*sweet potato "pie"
	herb tea

1,485

MENU 66

Calories	**BREAKFAST**
50	½ c orange juice
150	2 slices raisin wheat toast
45	1 tsp butter or margarine
140	1 c lowfat milk
	coffee or tea

SNACK

| 95 | 2 dates and 6 walnuts |

LUNCH

320	meat loaf sandwich (2 slices whole grain bread and 3 oz meat loaf)
5	lettuce and tomato
50	¾ c shredded carrot-apple salad
10	1 tbsp yogurt dressing
140	1 c lowfat milk

DINNER

240	*vegetable lasagna
140	2 slices garlic bread
45	1 tsp butter or margarine
25	tossed green salad
5	1 tbsp cucumber dressing
50	½ c grapefruit sections with kiwi fruit

1,510

MENU 67

Calories

BREAKFAST

50	½ grapefruit
140	1½ c shredded wheat
50	½ c peach slices
140	1 c lowfat milk
	coffee or tea

LUNCH

190	*3 oz oven-"fried" chicken
180	2 small corn muffins
45	1 tsp butter or margarine
20	marinated green bean salad
3	1 tbsp Lo-Cal tomato dressing
140	1 c lowfat milk
50	2 plums

DINNER

180	3 oz lean roast pork
50	½ c applesauce
135	cottage baked potato (1 small potato sliced and 1 tsp butter)
70	½ c green peas
20	mixed vegetable salad
45	1 tbsp ginger dressing

1,508

MENU 68

Calories	BREAKFAST
50	½ c orange juice
140	2 small whole grain rolls
45	1 tsp butter or margarine
20	2 tsp sugar-reduced jam
140	1 c lowfat milk
	coffee or tea

Calories	LUNCH
300	deluxe tuna sandwich (2 slices wheat bread, 3 oz tuna)
15	1 tbsp lemon-Dijon dressing,
15	sprouts, tomatoes, and
45	⅛ avocado)
140	1 c lowfat milk
50	2 apricots

Calories	DINNER
310	*3 oz lamb with artichokes
15	mixed green salad
10	1 tbsp buttermilk dressing
190	*2 sweet cheese crepes

1,485

MENU 69

Calories	BREAKFAST
50	1 orange, sectioned
80	1 egg omelet with tomatoes
70	1 potato, hashed
45	1 tsp butter or margarine
70	1 slice whole wheat toast
10	1 tsp sugar-reduced jam
140	1 c lowfat milk
	coffee or tea

LUNCH

30	1 c vegetable soup
300	grilled cheese sandwich (2 slices wheat bread, and 2 oz lowfat cheese)
45	1 tsp butter or margarine
20	*broccoli combination salad
140	1 c lowfat milk
50	½ banana

DINNER

165	½ small roasted Cornish hen with herbs
140	1 c whole wheat pasta with parsley sauce
20	steamed carrots, cauliflower, and zucchini
15	mixed green salad
45	1 tbsp French dressing
50	1 peach

1,475

MENU 70

Calories	BREAKFAST
50	½ c orange juice
140	⅓ c oatmeal, uncooked
50	2 tbsp dried fruit
140	1 c lowfat milk
	coffee or tea

LUNCH

330	bean tacos (2 corn tortillas, ½ c cooked beans, 1 oz cheese, and chili sauce)
20	fresh spinach salad
45	1 tbsp herb dressing
140	1 c lowfat milk
50	1 pear

DINNER

230	*beef curry
140	1 c steamed brown rice
20	mixed green salad
45	1 tbsp vinaigrette dressing
65	¾ c tangelo sections with 1 tbsp port wine

1,465

MENU 71

Calories	BREAKFAST
50	½ c orange juice
140	1 whole wheat English muffin
45	1 tsp butter or margarine
20	2 tsp sugar-reduced jam
140	1 c lowfat milk
	coffee or tea

Calories	LUNCH
275	salmon salad nicoise (3 oz salmon, 1 small potato, green beans, lettuce, and tomatoes)
45	1 tbsp herb dressing
70	1 small French roll
140	1 c lowfat milk
100	1 small banana

Calories	DINNER
325	*2 white bean steaks
20	steamed crookneck squash
15	mixed green salad
45	1 tbsp honey-mustard dressing
50	1 peach

1,480

MENU 72

Calories	BREAKFAST
50	½ c pineapple/grapefruit juice
140	⅓ c oatmeal, uncooked
50	2 dates, chopped
140	1 c lowfat milk
	coffee or tea

Calories	LUNCH
30	1 c vegetable soup
190	2 oz beef and 1 oz cheese
140	2 slices rye bread

15	sliced tomatoes, lettuce
45	1 tsp mayonnaise
140	1 c lowfat milk
50	1 pear

DINNER

180	3 oz baked chicken with herbs and wine
70	½ c rice pilaf
70	½ c green peas
45	1 tsp butter or margarine
25	cabbage and carrot slaw
45	1 tbsp vinaigrette dressing
50	baked apple

1,475

MENU 73

Calories   **BREAKFAST**

50	½ grapefruit
150	2 slices raisin wheat toast
45	1 tsp butter or margarine
140	1 c lowfat milk
	coffee or tea

LUNCH

180	3 oz lamb and shredded vegetables
140	whole wheat pita bread
30	shredded cucumber in yogurt-dill dressing
140	1 c lowfat milk
50	1 tangelo

DINNER

245	*beef stuffed acorn squash
70	1 small roll
45	1 tsp butter or margarine
20	endive and watercress salad
45	1 tbsp French dressing
155	*flan (caramel custard)

1,505

MENU 74

Calories	**BREAKFAST**
50	½ c orange juice
140	1½ c shredded wheat
25	1 tbsp raisins
140	1 c lowfat milk
	coffee or tea

	LUNCH
360	turkey salad on wheat bun (3 oz turkey, celery, onion, 1 tsp mayonnaise, and 2 tsp yogurt)
20	mixed green salad
45	1 tbsp vinaigrette dressing
140	1 c lowfat milk
50	½ banana

	DINNER
180	3 oz oven-"fried" pork chops
140	1 c tangy baked beans (white beans, tomato sauce, onion, mustard, and vinegar)
20	steamed broccoli
45	1 tsp butter or margarine
70	shredded carrot salad with 1 tsp mayonnaise
50	2 plums

1,475

MENU 75

Calories	**BREAKFAST**
50	½ c orange juice
210	2 slices French toast (2 slices whole wheat bread and 1 egg)
90	2 tsp butter
30	1 tbsp sugar-reduced syrup
140	1 c lowfat milk
	coffee or tea

LUNCH

105	¾ c pea soup
25	mixed vegetable salad
45	1 tbsp herb dressing
120	½ c lowfat cottage cheese
140	1 c lowfat milk
50	1 c melon cubes

DINNER

180	3 oz broiled steak with mushrooms
70	½ c golden whipped potatoes
25	stewed green beans with tomatoes
20	romaine lettuce salad
45	1 tbsp ginger dressing
132	*cranberry cake

1,477

MENU 76

Calories

BREAKFAST

50	½ c grapefruit juice
140	½ c Grape Nuts
50	½ c peach slices
140	1 c lowfat milk
	coffee or tea

LUNCH

380	bean and cheese burrito (1 flour tortilla, ⅓ c beans, 1½ oz lowfat cheese, and 1 tsp butter)
15	lettuce and tomatoes
45	⅛ avocado
140	1 c lowfat milk
50	½ c fruit cocktail

DINNER

250	*½ stuffed Cornish hen
20	steamed brussel sprouts
70	1 roll
45	1 tsp butter or margarine
70	berry parfait (⅔ c berries, and 2 tbsp yogurt)

1,465

MENU 77

Calories	BREAKFAST
50	½ c orange juice
140	2 slices wheat toast
90	2 tsp butter or margarine
20	2 tsp sugar-reduced orange marmalade
140	1 c lowfat milk
	coffee or tea

	LUNCH
165	3 oz tuna on salad greens
35	1 tbsp green goddess dressing
140	1 med French roll
45	1 tsp butter or margarine
140	1 c lowfat milk
50	2 figs

	DINNER
200	3 oz steak with shallots and chives
140	1 large oven-baked potato
45	1 tsp butter or margarine
35	sliced cucumbers in dill-yogurt dressing
50	½ mango

1,485

MENU 78

Calories	BREAKFAST
50	½ pink grapefruit
140	⅓ c whole wheat cereal, uncooked
140	1 c lowfat milk
25	1 tbsp raisins
	coffee or tea

	LUNCH
240	spinach and cheese omelet (1 egg and 2 oz lowfat cheese)
140	2 slices whole wheat bread

90	2 tsp butter or margarine
20	sliced tomatoes
140	1 c lowfat milk
50	1 apple

DINNER

185	*chicken Tandoori style (3 oz)
160	*1 c pilaf Indienne
20	mixed green salad
45	1 tbsp ginger dressing
50	½ c fresh fruit compote

1,495

MENU 79

Calories

BREAKFAST

50	½ grapefruit
150	2 slices raisin wheat toast
90	1 tbsp peanut butter
140	1 c lowfat milk
	coffee or tea

LUNCH

300	pasta salad (1 c pasta, 2 oz julienne meat or cheese, and assorted vegetables)
45	1 tsp mayonnaise
10	1 tbsp plain lowfat yogurt
140	1 c lowfat milk
50	1 apple

DINNER

260	*easy moussaka (beef and eggplant casserole)
140	1 c rice pilaf
20	tossed green salad
45	1 tbsp vinaigrette dressing
50	¼ melon

1,490

MENU 80

Calories	**BREAKFAST**
50	½ c orange juice
70	1 egg, scrambled
140	2 small potatoes, hashed
90	2 tsp butter or margarine
140	1 c lowfat milk
	coffee or tea

	LUNCH
200	turkey-barley soup (2 oz turkey, ½ c barley, and vegetables)
55	carrot-raisin salad (1 large carrot, 1 tbsp raisins, and 1 tbsp plain lowfat yogurt)
70	1 small roll
45	1 tsp butter or margarine
140	1 c lowfat milk
50	2 plums

	DINNER
170	*sea bass plaki
140	1 c steamed brown rice
20	spinach with lemon
100	*spicy stuffed pear

1,480

**BEEF
VEAL
PORK**

SHEPHERD'S BEEF AND POTATO PIE

13 oz round steak, thinly sliced (or 10 oz cooked roast
    beef)
1 onion, sliced
2 carrots, diced
1 rib celery, diced
½ c frozen peas, defrosted
½ c mushrooms, sliced
¼ c tomato puree
¼ c red wine
garlic powder
pepper
¼ tsp thyme
2 c mashed potatoes
2 oz lowfat cheese, shredded

Brown meat with its own juices in a large skillet.
Add onion, carrots, celery, peas, mushrooms, and tomato puree. Add seasoning to taste. Cook for about 20
minutes until vegetables are tender, but not mushy.
Add wine. Prepare mashed potatoes. Place meat mixture onto a casserole dish. Top with shredded cheese
and, then, the mashed potatoes. Bake uncovered until
potatoes are lightly browned (for about 25 minutes) at
350°F.

Makes 4 servings at 290 calories per serving.

BEEF STROGANOFF

1 lb beef round steak
1 leek, chopped
¼ c celery, chopped
2 tbsp carrots, shredded
½ c tomato, chopped
1 c mushrooms, sliced

1 c water
⅓ c dry white wine
1 tsp pepper
½ tsp garlic powder
2 tsp arrowroot
½ c plain lowfat yogurt

Cut round steak into cubes. Brown in its own juices. Add leeks, celery, carrots, and cook for 5 minutes. Add tomato, water, wine, garlic, and pepper. Simmer for 20 minutes. Add mushrooms and cook for 5 minutes longer. With some of the liquid from the sauce, dilute the arrowroot and stir into the mixture. Cook until thickened. Before serving, stir in yogurt. Serve over noodles.

Makes 4 servings at 240 calories per serving.

STIR-"FRIED" BEEF AND VEGETABLES

1 lb round steak, cut into strips
1 tbsp oil
1 med onion, thinly sliced
2 tbsp minced ginger root
¼ lb broccoli, broken into flowerets
½ lb celery, sliced
¼ lb snow peas
1 c Napa cabbage, shredded
½ c water
¼ c mushrooms, sliced
1 c bean sprouts
1 tbsp salt-reduced soy sauce

Sauté the meat in the oil until it loses its pinkness. Add onions and cook until they become transparent. Add ginger root, broccoli, celery, snow peas, cabbage, and water. Steam for 2 minutes or until vegetables are tender but crisp. Add mushrooms and sprouts and soy sauce. Cook for about 1 more minute, stirring to mix the soy sauce. May substitute turkey, chicken, pork, or shellfish.

Makes 4 servings. If using beef or pork, 270 calories per serving; if using turkey, chicken, or shellfish, 225 calories per serving.

SICILIAN VEAL WITH PASTA

1 lb veal, cut into 1-inch cubes
½ c green pepper, chopped
½ c onion, chopped
2 cloves garlic, minced
5 tomatoes, peeled and chopped
½ c sliced pitted olives
2 tbsp capers, drained
1 tsp dried basil, crushed
½ tsp oregano, crushed
½ tsp ground pepper
1½ c mushrooms, sliced

In a large skillet or Dutch oven, lightly brown the veal cubes in their own juice. Remove the veal and set aside. Into the pan, add the green peppers, onions, and garlic, and cook until vegetables are tender. Stir in chopped tomatoes, olives, capers, basil, oregano, and pepper. Simmer uncovered for about 15 minutes. Add the veal and cook for another 5 minutes or until sauce is slightly thickened and tomatoes are tender.

Makes 4 servings at 340 calories per serving, which includes 1 cup of cooked pasta per serving (pasta is 140 calories per cup).

SUKIYAKI

14 oz beef round steak
½ lb tofu (bean curd)
½ lb transparent noodles
10 slender green onions
½ lb Chinese or Savoy cabbage or bokchoy
6 dried Japanese mushrooms (Shitake mushrooms)
1 tbsp sesame seed oil
3 tbsp soy sauce, salt-reduced type
2 tbsp saké or dry sherry
1 tsp fructose
½ c chicken stock, double strength

Partially freeze steak to facilitate slicing. Slice into ⅛ inch slices. Set aside. Slice tofu into ½ inch slices and place under broiler until each side is golden. Set aside. Place noodles in boiling water until tender. Drain and set aside. Slice onions into 2 inch lengths. Cut cabbage into large pieces. Soak mushrooms in warm water for 20 minutes. On a large platter, arrange the steak, tofu, noodles, and vegetables in separate sections. Add the oil to a large skillet (nonstick). Put in the beef, a few pieces at a time, and brown lightly over medium heat. Add the tofu, noodles, onions, cabbage, and mushrooms to the skillet. Combine the soy sauce, sherry, fructose, and soup stock and sprinkle over the ingredients in the pan. Cook over medium heat until the vegetables are still firm. Sukiyaki may be cooked in an electric skillet on the table.

Makes 4 servings at 250 calories per serving.

LAMB WITH ARTICHOKES

1 tbsp olive oil
1 c chopped onion
1 garlic cloved minced
2 c frozen artichoke hearts
2 c sliced mushrooms
1½ c water
1 tbsp tomato paste
2 tbsp dry red wine
1 tbsp lemon juice
4 lamb chops, 5–6 oz each with bone

Sauté onion and garlic in oil until onion is transparent. Add artichoke hearts, mushrooms, water, tomato paste, wine, and lemon juice. Broil chops on rack for about 2 minutes on each side. Transfer chops to a baking dish. Top with artichoke mixture. Bake at 350°F for 20 minutes.

Makes 4 servings at 310 calories per serving.

SAVORY BEEF ROLL

2 lb round steak or flank steak
2 tbsp soy sauce, sodium-reduced
¼ c lemon juice
1 c onion, chopped
2 tbsp water
2 cloves garlic
½ c celery, chopped
½ c parsley, chopped

1 c mushrooms, chopped
½ tsp thyme
1 tsp black pepper
1 bay leaf
½ c red wine
2 c water or beef broth
½ c tomato puree

Pound steak to ½-inch thickness. Sprinkle with soy sauce and lemon juice. Marinate for 2 hours.

In a saucepan, sauté onions and garlic in water until transparent. Add celery, parsley, and mushrooms and cook for 10 minutes over low heat. Stir in thyme and pepper.

Place steak on a sheet pan and evenly distribute vegetable mixture over steak. Roll in jelly roll fashion, using a string to tie it together. Place in a large pot to which bay leaf, wine, water, and tomato puree have been added. Simmer for 40 minutes, covered. Allow to cool slightly before slicing.

Makes 8 servings at 210 calories per serving.

CORNBREAD-TOPPED BEEF AND CHILI CASSEROLE

1½ lb round steak
1 onion, minced
1 clove garlic
2 c cooked kidney beans, drained
½ c green California chili, chopped
⅔ c tomato puree
¾ c water
1 c beer
1 tbsp chili powder

CORNBREAD TOPPING

¾ c corn meal
1 c flour
1 tbsp butter
1½ tsp baking powder
1 egg
⅔ c lowfat milk

Slice the steak into thin strips. In a large non-stick skillet, sauté the steak with the onions and garlic. Cook until onions are transparent. Add the kidney beans, chili, tomato puree, water, beer, and chili powder. Simmer together for about 20 minutes. Meanwhile, prepare the cornbread topping. Mix the corn meal and flour with the butter. Add the baking powder. Beat the egg and mix with the milk. Add this to the dry ingredients and mix until the particles are moistened. Pour beef and chili mixture into a 2-quart casserole dish. Spread the cornbread topping over the mixture. Bake in a 350°F oven for about 25 minutes or until cornbread is golden brown.

Makes 8 servings at 325 calories per serving.

EASY MOUSSAKA

1 med eggplant, sliced ½" thick
12 oz leanest ground beef
1 onion, chopped
½ c parsley, chopped
1 clove garlic, minced
1 large fresh tomato, chopped
¼ c red wine
2 tbsp chopped green pepper
2 tbsp chopped celery
scant ⅛ tsp cinnamon
4 oz shredded mozarella cheese

Steam eggplant slices for about 5 minutes until tender, but still firm. Set aside. Sauté ground beef with the onions until red from meat disappears. Add parsley, tomato, green pepper, celery, and garlic. Simmer for 25 minutes. Add wine and cinnamon.

Arrange half the eggplant slices in a casserole dish to make bottom layer. Spread meat sauce over eggplant. Add remaining eggplant layer. Sprinkle with mozarella cheese. Bake at 350°F for 25 to 30 minutes. May brown under broiler for last few minutes if desired.

Makes 4 servings at 260 calories per serving.

STEFADO GREEK (BEEF AND ONION) STEW

1 lb lean sirloin steak or flank or round steak
2 c tomatoes, peeled and chopped
1 lb small boiling onions

1 clove garlic
bay leaf
1 tsp whole pickling spice
½ c red wine
1 tsp pepper
¼ lb feta cheese, cubed
¼ c walnuts, coarsely chopped

Cut meat into small chunks. Brown in their own juices. Add tomatoes and simmer for 20 minutes. Peel onions and leave whole, and add to stew. Place garlic, bay leaf, and spices in a clean cheesecloth. Add this plus wine to mixture. Add a small amount of water as liquid becomes reduced. Cook tightly covered until onions are tender, for about 30 minutes. Before serving, toss feta cheese cubes and walnuts into stew.

Makes 4 servings at 230 calories per serving.

BEEF CURRY

1 lb round steak, thin strips
2 green apples, sliced and halved
½ large bellpepper, cubed
¾ c celery, finely chopped
1 onion, sliced
1 clove garlic, minced
2 carrots, cut diagonally into coins
2 tsp butter or margarine
1½ tbsp cornstarch
1½ c beef broth
2 tsp curry powder
cayenne pepper to taste
1 cinnamon stick

Cook onion and garlic over low heat to steam. Cook until onion is clear. Then add all other vegetables and sliced apples. Cook until tender but still firm.

In another pan cook beef strips in their own juice for about 5 minutes. Add to vegetable mixture.

Prepare sauce by mixing cornstarch with ¼ cup of the cold broth in a small saucepan. Stir well; then add remaining broth. Place over heat, stirring constantly. Add butter, curry, cinnamon stick, and pepper. Cook until thickened and bubbly. Pour over meat and vegetable mixture and gently simmer a few more minutes, stirring occasionally.

Makes 4 servings at 230 calories per serving.

BEEF-STUFFED ACORN SQUASH

2 med acorn squash
12 oz ground beef, very lean
½ c onion, chopped
¼ c celery, chopped
1 clove garlic, minced
½ c green peas
¼ tsp cinnamon
¼ tsp allspice
¼ tsp pepper

Cut the squash in half and remove seeds. Steam squash until tender when forked, for about 20 minutes. In the meantime, in a large nonstick skillet, sauté the beef, onion, and garlic until well browned. Stir in the seasoning and the peas. Remove the steamed squash and pack beef mixture firmly into the squash. You may need to enlarge the squash cavity by spooning out some pulp. Place in a shallow baking dish and bake for about 25 minutes at 350°F.

Makes 4 servings at 245 calories per serving.

BEEF AND RICE-STUFFED TOMATOES

8 med tomatoes
¾ lb leanest ground beef
1 med onion, chopped
1 clove of garlic, minced
¼ c parsley, chopped
1 tbsp mint, chopped
¾ c raw rice
1½ c water
¼ c tomato puree
2 tbsp currants or finely chopped raisins

Scoop out the pulp of each of the tomatoes, reserving both the pulps and the caps. Brown the meat, add the onion and the garlic, and cook until onion becomes transparent. Add parsley, mint, currants, rice, 1 cup of water, tomato puree, and tomato pulp. Simmer for 15 minutes. Fill each tomato equally with the mixture and cover with caps. Arrange in a baking pan and add the rest of the water. Bake at 350°F for about 25 minutes, basting occasionally.

Makes 4 servings at 240 calories per serving.

VEAL PARMESAN

14 oz veal round steak or veal cutlets
1 tsp margarine
½ c onion, sliced
½ c green pepper, sliced
¾ c tomatoes, chopped
½ tsp garlic powder
1 tsp dried basil
¼ c dry white wine
2 oz lowfat mozarella cheese, shredded
1 tbsp Parmesan cheese, grated

In a small skillet, sauté onions and green pepper in margarine. Add tomatoes, herbs, and wine. Simmer for 15 minutes.

With a mallet, pound veal steaks until they are ¼-inch thick. In a large nonstick skillet, lightly brown both sides of the veal. Place veal in a single layer on a baking pan. Cover with tomato sauce. Sprinkle with cheese. Bake in a 450°F oven for 10 minutes or until cheese melts.

Makes 4 servings at 220 calories per serving.

LINGUINE WITH EGGPLANT AND VEAL SAUCE

4 c cooked linguine
8 oz ground veal
1 clove garlic, minced
½ onion, chopped
2 c tomato puree
½ med eggplant, peeled and diced
½ green pepper, chopped
2 tbsp parsley, chopped
1 c fresh mushrooms, chopped
¼ c dry red wine
1 bay leaf

½ tsp dried oregano
½ tsp dried basil
½ tsp pepper
4 oz lowfat cheese, shredded

Sauté meat until lightly browned. Add garlic and onions. Continue to sauté for a few minutes longer. Add all ingredients except for the cheese. Simmer for 30 minutes. Add the herbs. Serve over hot linguine. Top each serving with 1 ounce of cheese.

Makes 4 servings at 245 calories per serving (include an additional 140 calories per cup of linguine).

PORK AND BEAN BAKE

2⅔ c cooked cannellini beans (may use great white
    northern beans)
*12 oz pork, lean, ground
1 onion, chopped
1 tsp oil
2 cloves garlic, minced
1½ c tomatoes, chopped
¼ tsp sage
¼ tsp oregano
¼ tsp basil
½ tsp pepper

Sauté onion and garlic in oil until slightly golden. Add pork and brown. Stir in tomatoes, beans, herbs, and spices. Pour into 4 individual oven-proof dishes. Bake uncovered at 350°F for 45 minutes.

Makes 4 servings at 275 calories per serving.

---

*Note: For leanest pork, ask your butcher to grind a well-trimmed pork roast.

HOMEMADE PORK SAUSAGE

1 lb lean pork, ground
3 tbsp parsley, chopped
½ tsp cloves
2 tsp sage
2 tsp ground pepper
1 tsp minced garlic
½ tsp oregano

Mix all ingredients. Shape into 12 patties. Place on baking sheet. Bake in a 400°F oven for about 20 minutes. Makes 12 servings at 70 calories per serving.

CHICKEN

CANTONESE CHICKEN

2 whole chicken breasts (10 oz each)
1 tsp sesame oil
½ c green onions
1 clove garlic, minced
1 tsp ginger, minced
½ c water chestnuts, sliced
½ c bamboo shoots
2 tsp soy sauce, sodium-reduced
1 tbsp cornstarch
1 c chicken broth
½ tsp red pepper

Skin and bone chicken breasts and cut into large cubes. Brown lightly in sesame oil. Add onions, garlic, and ginger. Simmer for 5 minutes. Add water chestnuts, bamboo shoots, and soy sauce. Mix cornstarch into ¼ cup of the chicken broth. Blend until smooth. Add to chicken mixture with remaining broth. Cook, stirring frequently until mixture thickens. Stir in red pepper.
Makes 4 servings at 180 calories per serving.

CHICKEN FLORENTINE

4 chicken breast halves, skinned
1½ c water
1 onion, chopped
2 cloves garlic
1 sprig parsley
1 bay leaf
1 tsp thyme
2 tsp butter
2 c mushrooms, sliced
½ c celery, chopped
½ c green bellpepper, sliced

½ c red bellpepper, sliced
½ c milk
2½ tbsp flour
¼ c dry sherry
2 lb fresh spinach or 2, 10 oz frozen package
3 tbsp Parmesan cheese, grated

Simmer the chicken breast in water; add the onion and in a cheesecloth place the garlic cloves, parsley, bay leaf, and the thyme and add to the pot. Cook until the chicken is tender. Remove the chicken from the stock. Bone the chicken and cut into 1-inch cubes. Remove any fat and residue from the stock and reserve the stock. Meanwhile, wash the spinach and cook in ½ cup of the reserved stock.

In a saucepan, sauté the mushrooms, celery, and green and red peppers in 2 teaspoons of butter until vegetables are tender. Remove the vegetables and put aside. In the same saucepan, add the milk and stir in the flour until smooth. Add 1 cup of the cooled chicken stock and stir. Place on a low heat, stirring constantly until the sauce thickens and bubbles. To this, add the sautéed vegetables, the sherry, and the chicken cubes. Cook until all are thoroughly heated.

Arrange the cooked, drained spinach on a flame-proof serving platter. Cover with the chicken mixture and sprinkle with the Parmesan cheese. Place under a hot broiler to just brown the sauce before serving.

Makes 4 servings at 255 calories per serving.

CHICKEN COUSCOUS

2 chicken breasts, skinned and boned (8 oz each)
2 tsp margarine
1 clove garlic, minced
½ c onion, chopped
⅓ c green pepper, chopped
2 tomatoes, chopped
½ c zucchini, diced
⅓ c carrots, diced
¼ c parsley, chopped
⅓ c celery, chopped
½ c garbanzo beans
1 c water

⅛ tsp red pepper
½ tsp dill weed
½ tsp coriander
¼ tsp tumeric
4 c precooked couscous
4 c chicken stock

Cut each chicken breast in quarters. Lightly brown chicken breasts in margarine. Sauté onions and garlic. Add all other ingredients except for the couscous and the chicken stock. Simmer for 45 minutes. Add the spices in the last 10 minutes.

Prepare couscous as directed by its package, using chicken broth for the liquid. Use 1 cup couscous (cooked) and ½ chicken breast with ¼ of the vegetable mixture per serving.

Makes 4 servings at 350 calories per serving.

CHICKEN LIVERS PAYSANNE

1 med onion, chopped
2 tsp butter
1 lb chicken livers, cut into thirds
½ tsp marjoram
2 tbsp parsley, chopped
¼ c red wine
¼ c lowfat sour cream
¼ c plain lowfat yogurt
½ tsp white pepper

Sauté the onion in the butter. Add the chicken livers and cook for 5 minutes. Add the marjoram, parsley, and wine. Simmer for about 3 minutes. Then add the sour cream, yogurt, and pepper. Simmer on very low heat for about 5 minutes until sauce is thoroughly heated.

Makes 4 servings at 210 calories per serving.

CHICKEN TANDOORI STYLE

4 chicken breast halves, about 4 oz each, deboned and
   skinned
½ tsp cayenne pepper
2 tsp curry powder
2 cloves garlic, minced

½ tsp paprika
¼ c lemon juice
¼ c red wine vinegar
¾ c onions, chopped
¼ c pimento, chopped
¾ c plain lowfat yogurt
¼ tsp ground ginger

Pierce chicken pieces in several places with a sharp fork. Arrange pieces in a baking dish. Combine cayenne, curry, garlic, paprika, lemon juice, and vinegar. Pour over chicken covering each piece. Allow to marinate in the refrigerator for 1 hour.

In a blender, combine onions, pimento, yogurt, and ginger. Mix for 10 seconds on medium. Pour over chicken. Bake at 325°F for 45 minutes or until tender. Baste frequently while baking.

Makes 4 servings at 185 calories per serving.

CHICKEN AND SHRIMP EGG ROLLS

8 oz cooked chicken, shredded
5 tsp sesame seed oil
1 onion, chopped
1 clove garlic
2 c Chinese cabbage, shredded
½ c pea pods, chopped
½ c water chestnuts, chopped
6 oz cooked bay shrimp
1 egg, beaten
2 tbsp sherry
2 tsp soy sauce
red pepper to taste
sweet and sour sauce (see recipe below)
8 egg roll skins

In wok or nonstick skillet add 1 teaspoon of oil, and cook onion, garlic, and cabbage for 2 to 3 minutes. Add pea pods and water chestnuts. In a bowl, combine chicken, shrimp, egg, sherry, soy sauce, and cooked vegetables. Brush one side of each egg roll skin with ½ teaspoon of oil. On un-oiled side place 2 tablespoons of vegetable chicken mixture. Roll into cylinder, tucking in ends of egg roll. Place on a baking sheet and bake at

350°F for 15 to 20 minutes or until rolls are golden brown. Serve with sweet and sour sauce.

Makes 8 servings at 155 calories per serving.

SWEET AND SOUR SAUCE

2 tbsp frozen concentrated pineapple juice
2 tsp fructose
1 tbsp cornstarch
⅓ c red wine vinegar
⅓ c chicken broth
2 tbsp pimento, chopped
1 tbsp soy sauce
¼ tsp garlic powder
¼ tsp ginger powder

In a small saucepan combine cornstarch with cold chicken broth. Stir in remaining ingredients. Cook and stir over medium heat until thickened and bubbly. Serve warm.

Makes about 1 cup at 5 calories per tablespoon.

TURKEY KABOBS

1 lb turkey breast, raw, cut into cubes
10–12 cherry tomatoes
1 green bellpepper, chunked
⅔ c pineapple chunks
½ lb mushrooms

MARINADE

½ c red wine vinegar
2 tbsp tomato paste
¼ c water
¼ c pineapple juice, frozen concentrate, undiluted
1 tbsp oil
¼ tsp tarragon
1 onion sliced
1 minced garlic
pepper to taste

Prepare marinade. Marinate turkey cubes for 4 hours in refrigerator. Divide turkey cubes, tomatoes, bellpepper, pineapple, and mushrooms among each of 8 skewers. Place only 2 ounces of turkey on each skewer. Alternate turkey with the various vegetables. Cook kabobs over hot coals for about 10 minutes, or broil 4 inches from flame for 8 to 10 minutes, turning kabobs as they brown and basting with reserved marinade.

Makes 8 kabobs or 4 servings at 190 calories per serving.

MEXICAN CHICKEN AND CHEESE CASSEROLE

¾ c raw brown rice
2½ c chicken broth
2 whole chicken breasts (8–9 oz each)
2 cloves garlic, minced
1 onion, chopped
1 red bellpepper sliced, or ½ c pimento, sliced
½ c California green chile
2 tomatoes, peeled and chopped
½ tsp red pepper
4 oz lowfat cheese, shredded
¼ c cilantro (fresh coriander), chopped

Cook rice in broth until rice is slightly underdone.

Divide whole chicken breasts into halves; remove skin and bone. Brown lightly in nonstick skillet. Add garlic and onion and cook until golden. Add red bellpepper, green chile, and tomatoes. Cover and simmer for 10 minutes.

Arrange chicken breasts in a baking dish, saving vegetables. Mix vegetables with rice and pour over chicken. Sprinkle with cheese. Bake for 25 minutes at 350°F. Sprinkle with cilantro before serving if desired.

Makes 4 servings at 340 calories per serving.

STUFFED CORNISH HEN

2 small Cornish hens (16–20 oz each)
1 tbsp water
⅓ c onion, chopped
2 tbsp celery, chopped
2 tbsp carrot, chopped
½ c buckwheat kernels (may also use brown rice)
1 c water or chicken broth
2 tbsp parsley, chopped

1 green apple, diced
½ tsp sage
¼ tsp thyme
¼ tsp pepper

In a medium-size saucepan, steam onions, celery, and carrots in the 1 tablespoon of water until tender. Add buckwheat kernels or brown rice, and water or chicken broth. Add parsley. Cook over low heat until grains are tender, for about 15 minutes for buckwheat, and for about 45 minutes for brown rice. Stir in apple, sage, thyme, and pepper. Divide stuffing into two equal portions and fill cavity of washed hens. Bake in a shallow baking pan at 350°F for about 45 minutes or until golden brown. To serve, remove skin and divide each hen in half. Serve half of the stuffing in each hen per person.

Makes 4 servings at 250 calories per serving.

HUNGARIAN CHICKEN

4 chicken breast halves, skinned and boned (4 oz each)
2 tsp margarine
1 med onion, thinly sliced
2 cloves of garlic, minced
1 med red or green pepper, sliced
1 c mushrooms, sliced
1 c chicken stock
2 tbsp white wine
¾ c plain lowfat yogurt
2 tsp arrowroot
2–3 tsp paprika

In a nonstick skillet, brown chicken in margarine. Add onions and garlic; cook until tender. Add peppers, mushrooms, and stock. Simmer covered for 25 minutes. Stir arrowroot into ¼ cup of the chicken stock until dissolved. Include mixture into skillet and stir until thickened. Add paprika to taste. Mix yogurt into skillet before serving. Do not boil after this point. Serve over rice.

Makes 4 servings at 165 calories per serving.

ROSEMARY CHICKEN

2 whole chicken breasts (8 oz each deboned and skinned)
3 tbsp whole wheat flour
1 tsp butter or margarine
1 clove garlic, minced
⅔ c green onions, sliced
1 c mushrooms, sliced
½ c white wine
1 tsp dried rosemary
1 tsp white pepper

Divide each chicken breast in half. Dust with the flour. In a large nonstick skillet over high heat, melt the butter and quickly brown the chicken breasts on each side with the garlic. Add onions, mushrooms, wine, rosemary, and pepper. Cover skillet with lid and simmer for about 20 minutes or until vegetables are tender.

Makes 4 servings at 180 calories per serving.

OVEN-FRIED CHICKEN

4 chicken breast halves, med
½ c lowfat milk
½ c plain dry bread crumbs
2 tsp butter, melted
½ tsp pepper
¼ tsp paprika
¼ tsp garlic powder
¼ tsp onion powder

Mix bread crumbs, butter, and seasonings. Remove skin from chicken. Dip the chicken into the milk; then roll into bread crumb mixture. Place them on a nonstick baking sheet and bake for 30 minutes in a 350°F oven.

Makes 4 servings at 190 calories per serving.

Note: May oven "fry" fish, substituting 1 beaten egg for the milk and 2 teaspoons of oil for the butter.

SEAFOOD

SEA BASS PLAKI

1 lb sea bass fillets, cut into 4 equal portions
1 c minced parsley
1 onion, thinly sliced
2–3 tomatoes, thinly sliced
1 clove garlic, minced
¼ c fresh lemon juice
½ tsp pepper

In a shallow baking pan spread half of the parsley. Lay the fillets on the parsley; season with the lemon juice, garlic, and pepper. Arrange onion slices over the fish, sprinkle with remaining parsley, and arrange tomato slices on top lastly. Bake in a 350°F oven for 35 minutes or until fish begins to flake when forked.

Makes 4 servings at 170 calories per serving.

ESCABÈCHE
(MARINATED FISH WITH VEGETABLES)

1 lb skinless, boneless fish fillets
2 tbsp lemon juice
1 med onion, thinly sliced
1 clove garlic, minced
2 small carrots, diced
2 small celery stalks, diced
1 tbsp olive oil
¼ c wine vinegar
1 tsp dried thyme
⅛ tsp pepper
1 bay leaf

Rinse fish in cold water and pat dry. Cut into 1-ounce pieces. Sprinkle with lemon juice. In a skillet, sauté the onions, carrots, celery, and garlic in the olive oil until vegetables are tender. Add the vinegar, thyme, pepper, and bay leaf and lower heat to a simmer. Carefully place the pieces of fish over the vegetable mixture and cover skillet tightly. Continue to cook for about 5 minutes if fish is ½-inch thick. (Cook 10 minutes if fish is 1-inch thick.) Remove contents from the pan and place onto a glass or ceramic dish and cover and refrigerate for at least 4 hours before serving. Garnish with lemon wedge, parsley, and lettuce leaves.

Makes 4 servings at 185 calories per serving.

SEVICHE
(MARINATED FRESH FISH)*

1 lb very fresh skinless, boneless fish fillets
    (flounder or sole or bass are good)
¼ c lime juice (may use lemon)
2 tbsp olive oil
1 tsp minced garlic
¾ c tomatoes, peeled and seeded, diced
2 tbsp parsley, finely chopped
2 tbsp fresh cilantro (coriander, fresh)
⅛ tsp crushed red pepper flakes
½ c green onions, finely chopped

Rinse the fish in cold water and pat dry. Cut into ¾-inch cubes and place in a bowl. Add all of the above ingredients except for the tomatoes and green onions. Refrigerate for at least 8 hours before serving. Before serving, stir in tomatoes and onions.

Makes 4 servings at 180 calories per serving.

*The acid from the lime juice "cooks" the fish.

BAKED SALMON WITH WINE AND
VEGETABLE SAUCE

1 lb salmon fillet
1 c dry white wine
2 carrots, neatly diced
1 celery stalk, neatly diced
1 onion, diced
1 tbsp butter
½ c lowfat milk
2 tbsp flour
1 tbsp chives, chopped
1 tbsp parsley, chopped
1 tbsp dried tarragon, crushed
dash of white pepper

Place fish in a baking dish, pouring the wine on top. Bake in a 350°F oven, basting with the wine. The fish should be done in about 15 minutes, depending on thickness. Do not overcook; fish is done when it feels springy to the touch. Remove from the oven and drain juices into a saucepan; cover the fish and keep it warm.

While the fish is baking, sauté the carrots, celery, and onions with the butter. Cook until the vegetables are tender, but not browned. Into the saucepan with the fish juices, add the milk into which the flour was added to have made a smooth paste. Stir over a medium heat until the sauce is thickened and bubbly. (This sauce will not be too thick.) Stir in the sautéed vegetables, the chives, parsley, and tarragon and pepper. Cook on a low heat to thoroughly heat all ingredients.

Place the fish on an attractive oblong platter, and pour the sauce over. Garnish with extra chopped chives and parsley.

Makes 4 servings at 220 calories per serving.

MAGIC CRUST SHRIMP PIE

6 oz baby shrimp
1 c lowfat cheddar cheese, shredded
½ c lowfat mozarella cheese, shredded
¼ c green onions, sliced
¼ c pimento, chopped
2 tbsp parsley, chopped
2 c buttermilk
4 eggs
1 c flour, unbleached
2 tbsp butter
½ tsp baking powder
½ tsp baking soda

Combine shrimp, cheeses, onions, pimento, and parsley in a lightly greased and floured 10 x 1½-inch pie plate. Place remaining ingredients in a blender. Blend at high speed for 15 seconds. Pour over ingredients in a pie plate. Bake in a 350°F oven for 35 to 40 minutes or until a knife inserted in the center comes out clean. Cool for 5 minutes before serving.

Makes 6 servings at 350 calories per serving, or 8 servings at 265 calories per serving.

SEAFOOD KABOBS

1 lb thick fish fillets or scallops or prawns
juice of 2 lemons
3 garlic cloves, minced
3 tbsp parsley, minced
2 tsp oregano
1 tbsp oil
¼ c white wine
½ tsp white pepper

Cut fish into 1½-inch cubes. Place all other ingredients in a bowl, add seafood, and mix well. Marinate for at least 1 hour. String the seafood equally among 4 skewers. Place on a broiler rack with a pan underneath to catch the drippings. Pour marinade over them and broil, basting and turning occasionally until they are golden on all sides.

Makes 4 servings at 165 calories per serving.

CIOPPINO

8 oz fresh or frozen fish fillets
4 oz shrimp, shelled and deveined
4 oz clams, chopped
¼ c onion, chopped finely
⅓ large green pepper, chunked
1 clove garlic, minced
2 tsp olive oil
2 c tomatoes, peeled, seeded, and chopped
4 oz tomato puree
½ c water
¼ c dry white wine
2 tbsp parsley, snipped
⅛ tsp each thyme and rosemary
pepper to taste

Remove any skin from fish fillets. Cut into 1-inch pieces. In a large nonstick skillet, cook onions, green pepper, and garlic in the oil until the onion is tender but not browned. Add tomatoes, tomato puree, water, parsley, thyme, rosemary, and pepper. Simmer covered for about 20 minutes. Then add fish pieces, shrimp, and clams to tomato mixture. Bring just to boiling then reduce heat and simmer covered for 5 to 7 minutes or until fish and shrimp are done. (Do not overcook fish; if using canned clams, add during the last 2 minutes of cooking.)

Makes 4 servings at 195 calories per serving.

POLYNESIAN FISH

4 4–oz fish fillets
2 tbsp vinegar
¼ c pineapple juice concentrate, undiluted
2 tbsp soy sauce, sodium-reduced
1 tsp oil
½ tsp ground ginger

Mix vinegar, juice, soy sauce, oil, and ginger. Let fish stand for 10 minutes in this sauce. Arrange fish in a broiler pan and broil about 4 inches from the heat source for 10 minutes or until fish flakes. Baste once during the broiling time with the sauce in the pan.

Makes 4 servings at 170 calories per serving.

HALIBUT MARENGO

4 halibut steaks (4 oz each)
2 tomatoes, diced
1 c tomato juice
2 tbsp lemon juice
1 c mushrooms, sliced
½ c celery, diced
2 tbsp onion, minced
¼ tsp thyme
¼ tsp white pepper
2 tbsp parsley, chopped

Place halibut in a shallow baking dish. Into a saucepan, combine all ingredients except parsley. Simmer for about 10 minutes. Pour over the halibut. Bake uncovered at 375°F for 15 to 20 minutes or until fish begins to flake when tested with a fork. Garnish with parsley.

Makes 4 servings at 165 calories per serving.

CLAM RISOTTO

1⅓ c long grain brown rice
1½ c water

1½ c clam juice
1 tbsp butter or margarine
⅓ c thinly sliced leeks or onions
⅓ c frozen peas
¼ c sweet red pepper, chopped
¼ c thinly sliced celery
⅓ c tomatoes, peeled, seeded and chopped
⅓ c fresh mushrooms, quartered
12 oz clams, chopped
½ tsp thyme
1 tbsp parsley, snipped

In a medium-size saucepan, cook rice in the water for 15 minutes. Remove from heat and keep the lid on.

In a larger saucepan, cook leeks and red pepper in butter until tender. Stir in peas, celery, and partly cooked rice. Add the clam juice and simmer for 15 minutes. Stir in tomatoes, mushrooms, clams, and herbs. Simmer slowly for about 7 minutes.

Makes 4 servings at 340 calories per serving.

RED SNAPPER SAN DIEGO

4 red snapper fillets (4 oz each)
1 tsp margarine
½ c onions, thinly sliced
1 clove of garlic, minced
½ c green pepper or chili, diced
2 whole tomatoes, diced
½ c shredded mozarella cheese, lowfat
1 tbsp cilantro (optional)

Sauté onions, garlic, and green pepper (or chili) in margarine. Cook until onion is lightly browned. Add tomatoes and cook for 15 minutes longer.

Arrange fillets in a nonstick baking pan. Cover the fish with the mixture. Broil fish from about 4 inches under the heat source for about 10 minutes or until fish flakes when forked. Sprinkle with cheese and broil until cheese melts. Garnish with chopped cilantro.

Makes 4 servings at 230 calories per serving.

LAYERED COD AND SPINACH LOAF

1 lb cod fillet
½ c zucchini, grated
⅓ c onion, grated
1 c spinach, chopped and cooked
2 eggs, slightly beaten
½ c bread crumbs
¼ c Parmesan cheese, grated
1 tsp garlic powder
½ tsp white pepper
1 c sliced mushrooms
2 tbsp white wine

Arrange half of the cod fillets in the bottom of a
loaf pan. In a mixing bowl, mix all ingredients except
for the mushrooms and the wine. Place the mixture
over the cod fillets in the loaf pan. Cover with the
remaining cod fillets. Bake at 350°F for 45 minutes.
Before serving, sauté mushrooms in the wine and then
spoon over the cod. Serve with lemon wedges.

Makes 4 servings at 225 calories per serving.

SHRIMP-STUFFED PASTA SHELLS

20 pasta shells, king-size (*conchiglioni*)
1 onion, chopped
1 tbsp water
½ c celery, chopped finely
⅓ c parsley, chopped
2 c spinach, chopped, or 1 pkg. frozen spinach,
   defrosted and drained
1 egg
1 c lowfat cottage cheese
¼ c bread crumbs
1 tsp tarragon
1 tsp white pepper
1½ c bay shrimp, cooked

CHEESE SAUCE

½ c onions, thinly sliced
1 tsp water
4 tbsp cornstarch
2 c lowfat milk

½ c white wine
½ c shredded lowfat mozarella cheese
½ tsp white pepper

Cook pasta shells according to package directions until just tender. Drain. Rinse in cold water. Drain.

Meanwhile, sauté onion in water until transparent. Add celery, parsley, and spinach. Cook for about 6 minutes. In a small bowl, beat egg. Mix in cottage cheese, bread crumbs, tarragon, and pepper. Stir in cooked vegetables and shrimp. In a large baking dish, arrange pasta shells. Fill each evenly with shrimp mixture. Cover with cheese sauce. Cover with foil and bake in a 350°F oven for 25 minutes.

Cheese Sauce

Sauté onions in water until transparent. Stir cornstarch into ½ cup of the cold milk. Blend until smooth. Add to onions and stir in rest of milk. Cook until thickened, stirring constantly. Add cheese and blend. Add wine and white pepper.

Makes 4 servings at 335 calories per serving.

OYSTERS BIENVILLE STYLE

12 med raw oysters in shell
¼ c green onion, finely chopped
1 small clove garlic, minced
1 tsp butter
1 tbsp flour
⅓ c chicken broth
2 tbsp white wine
¼ c mushrooms, finely chopped
1 tbsp parsley, finely chopped
¼ c bread crumbs
2 tsp Parmesan cheese
1 tsp butter

Open oysters with knife and remove oysters. Wash shells. Arrange oysters on deep shell halves in a shallow baking dish. Use crumpled aluminum foil to keep shells upright, if necessary.

For sauce cook onion and garlic in butter until tender. Stir in flour and broth. Cook and stir until thickened and bubbly. Add wine, mushrooms, and parsley. Remove from heat. In a small bowl toss bread crumbs, Parmesan cheese, and butter.

Bake oysters in 400°F oven for 5 minutes. Top each oyster with 1 tablespoon of sauce. Sprinkle 1 teaspoon of crumb mixture over sauce. Bake at 400°F for an additional 10 to 12 minutes. Garnish with parsley sprig.

Makes 2 servings at 170 calories per serving.

Note: You may leave out butter to reduce calories by 45 calories per serving.

EXECUTIVE CRAB CASSEROLE

10 oz pkg artichoke hearts, frozen or canned
8 oz crab meat, chunked or flaked
1 c mushrooms, sliced
½ c onions, minced
1 tsp butter or margarine
2½ tbsp flour
1 c lowfat milk
1 tsp Worcestershire sauce
¼ c dry sherry
paprika to taste
cayenne pepper to taste
¼ c grated Parmesan cheese

Sauté onions and mushrooms in butter until lightly golden. Place artichokes in bottom of greased baking dish; spread a layer of crab meat over. Add a layer of mushrooms and onions. Add remaining ingredients except cheese in a saucepan, stirring well, over medium heat to form a smooth sauce. Pour sauce over artichoke-crab layers and sprinkle cheese on top. Bake at 375°F for 20 minutes.

Makes 4 servings at 200 calories per serving.

VEGETARIAN DISHES

VEGETABLE LASAGNA

1 eggplant, sliced lengthwise
2–3 zucchini, sliced lengthwise
3 tbsp flour
2–3 summer squash
1 onion, sliced
1 green pepper, sliced
1 clove garlic, minced
1 tsp olive oil
2 c tomatoes, peeled and chopped
½ tsp basil
½ tsp oregano
½ tsp black pepper
2 tbsp red wine
2½ c lowfat cottage cheese
1 egg
¼ c parsley, chopped
½ c green onion, chopped
½ c mozarella cheese, lowfat, grated
1 tbsp Parmesan cheese

Blanch eggplant, zucchini, and other squash until just tender when forked. Set aside. Sauté onion, green pepper, and garlic in the olive oil. Add tomatoes, basil, oregano, pepper, and wine. Simmer for 15 to 20 minutes; longer if tomatoes are fresh.

Meanwhile in a small bowl, beat egg; add the cottage cheese, parsley, and green onion. Set aside.

Take the blanched vegetables and dust each piece with the flour. Pour about ½ cup of the tomato sauce in the bottom of a shallow 1½-quart casserole dish. Arrange a layer of half the vegetables on top. Spread half of cottage cheese mixture over this layer. Repeat this layering process. Top with remaining tomato sauce. Sprinkle with mozarella cheese. Bake at 350°F for 1 hour.

Makes 4 servings at 240 calories per serving.

WHITE BEAN STEAKS

3 c cooked white beans (canellini or great northers)
1 c celery, chopped
1 c onion, chopped
1 clove garlic
1 tbsp oil
1 egg
¼ c parsley, chopped
¼ tsp basil
¼ tsp oregano
dash thyme
4 oz lowfat mozarella cheese, shredded

Sauté onions and garlic in 1 tablespoon of oil. Cook until transparent. Add celery and cook until tender. Meanwhile, mash beans until some large chunks of beans still remain. Add in onion mixture and all other ingredients except cheese. Form into 8 patties about ½ inch thick. Place on nonstick baking sheet. Bake at 350°F for about 20 minutes. Top each patty with ½ ounces of cheese and bake for an additional 10 minutes.

Makes 8 patties at 160 calories per serving.

VEGETABLE STRUDEL

1 onion, chopped
1 tsp oil
1 clove garlic
2 c spinach, chopped, or 10 oz package, defrosted, drained
2 c mustard greens, chopped, or 10 oz package, defrosted, drained
1 c parsley, chopped
1 c watercress
½ c mushrooms, chopped
1 c cottage cheese
½ tsp white pepper
¼ tsp nutmeg
½ tsp thyme
Filo (Greek pastry dough)
4 tsp butter or margarine

Sauté onion in oil; add garlic. Add spinach, mustard greens, watercress, and parsley. Simmer for 10 minutes, uncovered. Stir in mushrooms and cottage cheese, pepper, nutmeg, and thyme.

Melt butter in small saucepan. Place 2 sheets of filo on wax paper. (Reroll and cover filo with plastic wrap between layering process.) Brush with butter. Place another 2 filo on top; brush with butter. Repeat until 8 filo leaves are used. Spread vegetable mixture on narrow end of filo layers. Roll like a strudel, tucking sides inward to seal. Brush roll with remaining butter; place on a baking sheet. Bake at 350°F for 35 minutes or until golden brown.

Makes 4 servings at 160 calories per serving.

VEGETABLE CASSOULET

1 onion, chopped
1 garlic clove, minced
1 tbsp olive oil
1 lb spinach, cut into large pieces
2 carrots, shredded
1 c chopped tomatoes
½ lb mushrooms, sliced
½ tsp oregano
½ tsp basil
¼ tsp pepper
12 oz shredded mozarella cheese (part skim)
3½ c cooked white beans

Sauté garlic and onions in oil. Do not brown. Steam spinach until just wilted. Set aside. To the garlic and onion mixture add the carrots, tomatoes, mushrooms, and seasonings and cook for 10 minutes. Into a 2-quart, deep casserole, layer half of the beans, topped by a layer of half of the spinach, topped by a layer of half of the cheese and half of the vegetable sauce. Repeat the layers ending with the cheese on the top. Bake in a 350°F oven for 1 hour.

Makes 6 servings at 370 calories per serving.

LAYERED CHEESE ENCHILADAS

10 corn tortillas
1¼ c Mexican chile sauce (see recipe below)

8 oz mozarella cheese, lowfat, shredded
1 c green onions, chopped
½ c plain lowfat yogurt
2 tbsp lowfat sour cream

Dip each tortilla into heated chile sauce. Place 1 tortilla in a small, shallow, ungreased baking dish; spoon over surface about 2 tablespoons of shredded cheese, 2 tablespoons of chopped green onion, and a little of the chile sauce. Add remaining tortillas, preparing each layer the same way. Pour remaining sauce over the stack, and top with remaining cheese.

Bake uncovered in a 350°F oven for 15 to 20 minutes or until hot, and cheese on top is golden. Cut into 4 wedges to serve. May serve with a mixture of the yogurt and sour cream.

Makes 4 servings at 335 calories per serving without cream, or 360 calories with cream.

MEXICAN CHILE SAUCE

3 med size tomatoes, peeled and chopped
½ c diced California green chiles
¼ c minced onion
1 tbsp cilantro, snipped
1 tsp garlic, minced
½ tsp oregano
¼ tsp cumin

Place all sauce ingredients in a blender until smooth. Transfer to a saucepan and simmer uncovered for 10 minutes, for flavors to blend.

SPINACH-CHEESE PIE (SPANOKOPETA)

2 bunches of spinach, cleaned and dried
¾ c lowfat cottage cheese
½ lb feta cheese, crumbled
2 eggs, beaten slightly
½ minced onion
¼ c chopped parsley
½ tsp dried dill weed
½ tsp pepper
½ c raw rice

CRUST

1 c whole wheat flour
1 c unbleached white flour
⅓ c margarine
¼ c water (enough to make a soft ball)

Place flour in a mixing bowl. Blend in margarine with a pastry blender until mixture is crumbly. Sprinkle with cold water. Mix with fork and roll mixture into a ball. Use a little more than ½ of the dough to cover the bottom of a 12″ x 7½″ baking dish. Bake bottom dough at 350°F for 10 minutes.

Tear spinach into small pieces. Add minced onion, cottage cheese, feta cheese, eggs, parsley, dill weed, rice, and pepper. Place mixture onto crust. Cover with the remaining dough. Bake at 350°F for 35 to 45 minutes, or until top crust is golden brown in the center.

Makes 6 servings at 340 calories per serving.

LIMA BEANS IN TOMATO SAUCE

1⅔ c dried large lima beans
1 med onion, sliced thinly
1 clove garlic, minced
1½ c crushed tomatoes, fresh or canned
1 tbsp oil
½ tsp oregano, crushed
pepper to taste

Rinse beans well. Soak beans overnight in 6 cups of water. Next day, without changing water, bring to a boil, then simmer until beans are just tender, for about 45 minutes. Meanwhile, sauté onion in the oil; cook until lightly browned. Add minced garlic and crushed tomatoes. Simmer for 15 minutes. Add cooked beans, oregano and pepper, and cook for an additional 20 minutes.

Makes 4 servings at 230 calories per 1 cup serving.

TOFU AND VEGETABLE BAKE

1 tsp butter or margarine
1 c mushrooms, sliced
½ c onion, chopped

1 garlic clove, minced
½ c brown rice, uncooked
¾ lb tofu, diced
1 c zucchini, sliced
1 c cauliflower, floweret flowers, blanched
1 c water
1 tbsp soy sauce, sodium-reduced
pepper to taste
4 oz mozzarella cheese, lowfat, shredded

Sauté onions, garlic, and mushrooms in the butter until onions are lightly golden. In the bottom of a shallow 2-quart casserole, place rice; top with mushroom-onion mixture, zucchini, cauliflower, and tofu. Mix soy sauce with water. Pour over casserole. Top with mozzarella cheese. Cover with foil and bake at 350°F for about 1 hour. Remove foil. Bake for another 5 to 10 minutes until cheese is golden.

Makes 4 servings at 320 calories per serving.

TARTE NIÇOISE

6 small tomatoes, ripe
¾ c shredded mozzarella cheese, part skim
1 tbsp minced onion
1 tsp basil
white pepper to taste
cayenne pepper to taste
7 black olives
¼ c green bellpepper, sliced

CUSTARD

3 eggs
1½ c lowfat milk
¼ c mozzarella cheese, part skim, shredded
2 tbsp Parmeson cheese
1 tbsp minced onion
¼ tsp white pepper

WHOLE WHEAT CRUST

1 c whole wheat flour
3 tbsp oil
⅓ c water

Place flour in a mixing bowl. Combine oil and milk and add to flour all at once. Mix with a pastry blender until mixture forms into a ball. Roll out dough between sheets of wax paper to a 12-inch circle. Line a 9 or 10-inch pie plate or quiche pan with the pastry. Pierce dough in several places with a fork. Bake at 450°F for 10 minutes. Cool before filling.

Sauté the onions in a few drops of water until transparent. Cut the tomatoes in half crosswise and gently squeeze to remove all the seeds. Steam the tomatoes gently until tender unless tomatoes are very ripe. In a small bowl, mix together the cheese, onion, basil, and white and cayenne pepper. Press the mixture into the tomato halves. Arrange the tomatoes in a circle around the tarte crust and one in the center. Prepare the custard by beating the eggs and milk together, adding the cheeses, onion, and pepper. Pour the custard into the tarte crust around the tomatoes and arrange the olives and green pepper slices decoratively on the custard. Bake on the middle shelf of a 350°F oven for 35 to 40 minutes or until set.

Makes 6 servings at 330 calories per serving, or 8 servings at 245 calories per serving.

SALADS AND VEGETABLES

BROCCOLI COMBINATION SALAD

½ lb broccoli spears
½ lb cauliflower
1 small red onion (Bermuda), sliced into rings
1 c mushrooms, sliced
⅓ c wine vinegar
½ tsp fructose
1 tsp oil
white pepper to taste
pinch of basil or tarragon

Break broccoli and cauliflower into flowerets.
In a nonstick skillet, add oil and sliced onions. Cook for 3 minutes. Add broccoli, cauliflower, mush-

rooms, and wine vinegar into which fructose and herbs have been added. Cover skillet and steam for 2 minutes until vegetables are very firm. Serve hot or cold.

Makes 4 to 6 servings at 20–25 calories per serving.

PASTA SALAD

1 c cooked shells or elbow macaroni
2 oz shredded chicken
1 oz shredded lowfat cheese
¼ c artichokes, quartered
1 tbsp red pepper chopped
2 tbsp carrots, shredded
½ c zucchini, thinly sliced
1 tbsp green onions, sliced
1 tsp mayonnaise
1 tbsp yogurt
white pepper to taste
pinch of tarragon or basil

Toss all ingredients lightly. Serve.
Makes 1 serving at 390 calories per serving.

STUFFED EGGPLANT (IMAM BAILDI)

2 small, long eggplants
2 onions, chopped
2 large tomatoes, peeled and chopped
2 cloves garlic, minced
2 tbsp parsley, chopped
1 tsp pepper
4 tsp olive oil

Split eggplants in half lengthwise. With a spoon, scoop out the inner pulp of each eggplant leaving a shell of about ¼-inch or slightly thicker. Chop the pulp and set aside.

Heat the oil in a skillet; then add the onion and garlic, cooking until transparent. Add the eggplant pulp, stirring often, along with tomatoes, parsley, and pepper. Continue cooking for 20 minutes. Spoon equal amounts of the mixture into eggplant shells.

Place the eggplant halves in a baking pan in which ½ inch of water has been added. Bake uncovered in a 350°F oven for 30 minutes.

Makes 4 servings at 60 calories per serving.

BROWN RICE PILAF

1 c raw brown rice
¼ c onion, chopped finely
2 tbsp parsley, minced
2½ c broth (chicken or beef)

Sauté onion in a nonstick pan until it starts to brown. Add parsley, broth, and rice. Bring to a boil. When rice starts to boil, reduce heat to the lowest possible level. Cover and simmer for 45 minutes.

Makes 4 cups at 140 calories per serving.

PILAF INDIENNE

1 c basmati or long grain brown rice
2 tsp butter
1 onion, sliced thinly
2 tsp curry powder
1 cinnamon stick
2½ c chicken stock
½ c frozen peas
⅓ c green onions, sliced thinly
¼ c seedless white raisins
1 tbsp slivered almonds

In a nonstick saucepan, sauté the onions in the butter until lightly golden. Add the rice and stir until onions and rice are golden brown. Add curry, cinnamon stick, and chicken stock. Stir and bring to a boil. Reduce the heat and simmer with a tight lid for 20 minutes if using basmati rice, and 40 minutes if using brown rice.

In the last 10 minutes of cooking, remove the cinnamon stick and place peas, green onions, and raisins on top of the rice. Do not stir. Replace the lid and continue cooking. Before serving, gently toss the rice with a long pronged fork. Garnish each serving with slivered almonds.

Makes 4 servings at 160 calories per serving.

SALAD DRESSINGS

LO-CAL TOMATO DRESSING

¾ c tomato juice
1 tbsp minced onion
1 tbsp lemon juice
1 tbsp minced parsley
1 clove garlic, minced
pepper to taste

Combine all ingredients and mix well.
Makes 1 cup at 3 calories per tablespoon.

HONEY-MUSTARD DRESSING

½ c wine vinegar or rice vinegar
2 tbsp lemon juice
⅓ c oil
1 tsp honey
1 tsp Dijon mustard
2 tsp chopped parsley
2 tsp minced onion
pepper to taste

Combine all ingredients into a blender. Mix well.
Makes 1 cup at 45 calories per tablespoon.

HERB DRESSING

⅓ c oil
⅓ c wine vinegar or rice vinegar
3 tbsp lemon juice
2 tbsp water
2 tsp chopped parsley
1 tsp basil
½ tsp oregano
½ tsp tarragon
1 clove garlic, minced

Mix ingredients in a blender or shake in a jar.
Makes 1 cup at 45 calories per tablespoon.

LEMON-DIJON DRESSING

½ c fresh lemon juice
½ c plain lowfat yogurt
1 tbsp oil
2 tsp Dijon mustard
½ tsp dried dill weed
½ tsp white pepper

Mix all ingredients and refrigerate for 1 hour before serving.

Makes 1 cup at 15 calories per tablespoon.

VINAIGRETTE DRESSING

⅓ c oil (olive preferred)
⅓ c wine vinegar or rice vinegar
⅓ c fresh lemon juice
pepper to taste

Combine ingredients in a blender or shake in a jar.

Makes 1 cup at 45 calories per tablespoon.

GINGER DRESSING

Use vinaigrette dressing adding:
1 tsp minced ginger
1 tsp honey

Combine all ingredients in a blender or shake in a jar.

Makes 1 cup at 45 calories per tablespoon.

BUTTERMILK DRESSING

¾ c buttermilk
2 tbsp fresh lemon juice
1 tsp red pepper flakes
1 tsp dried basil
1 clove garlic, minced

Combine all ingredients in a blender. Mix well. Allow to sit in refrigerator for 2 hours before using.

Makes 1 cup at 8 calories per tablespoon.

GREEN GODDESS DRESSING

⅔ c plain lowfat yogurt
¼ c mayonnaise
2 tbsp minced green onion
2 tbsp minced parsley
½ tsp white pepper
1 clove garlic, minced

Mix all ingredients in a blender until smooth.
Makes 1 cup at 35 calories per tablespoon.

CUCUMBER DRESSING

½ c shredded cucumber
½ c plain lowfat yogurt
1 clove garlic, minced
1 tbsp minced green onion
½ tsp dill weed
½ tsp white pepper

Combine all ingredients and mix well. Allow flavors to marry by refrigerating for 1 hour before using.
Makes 1 cup at 5 calories per tablespoon.

FRENCH DRESSING

¼ c tomato puree
¼ c wine vinegar or cider vinegar
¼ c lemon juice
¼ c oil
¼ tsp dry mustard
½ tsp fructose
pepper to taste

Combine all ingredients in a blender or shake in a jar.
Makes 1 cup at 45 calories per tablespoon.

SOUPS

ALBONDIGAS SOUP (MEATBALL SOUP)

1 lb ground turkey (may use lean beef)
¼ c whole wheat flour

1 egg
32 oz chicken or turkey broth
2 med onions, chopped
½ tsp red pepper flakes
2 carrots, sliced diagonally
1 zucchini, sliced
2 small ears of corn
¼ c fresh cilantro, chopped
1 lime

Combine turkey, flour, egg, and ¼ cup of the broth. In a large pot bring remaining broth, onions, and pepper to a boil. Reduce heat to low. Form turkey mixture into balls about 1½ inches in diameter; mixture yields about 24 balls. Drop balls into stock. Simmer uncovered for about 5 minutes. Spoon off any fat and foam that may have surfaced. Add carrots, zucchini, and corn cobs which have been cut into two pieces each. Simmer for about 20 minutes or until carrots are tender.

Ladle out four portions with equal numbers of meatballs in each bowl. Top each serving with cilantro and squeeze lime juice over all.

Makes 4 servings at 215 calories per serving.

LENTIL-SPINACH SOUP

½ c + 1 tbsp lentils, uncooked
6 c water
1 small onion, sliced
1 tsp oil
2 ribs celery, chopped
½ lb spinach, chopped
1 c tomatoes, peeled and seeded
½ tsp pepper
¼ tsp garlic powder

Wash lentils and soak for 4 hours. Sauté onions in oil until golden. Add lentils and remaining ingredients. Simmer for about 1 hour or until lentils are soft.

Makes 4 servings at 120 calories per serving.

CHEESE BROCCOLI SOUP

½ c onion, chopped
1½ c chicken broth

1 garlic clove
1 bay leaf
3 tbsp flour
1 c milk, lowfat
10 oz or 2 c broccoli, chopped
8 oz lowfat cheddar cheese, shredded
1 tbsp Worcestershire sauce

Add the onion, broth, garlic, and bay leaf to a medium-size saucepan and simmer until onion is transparent. Remove the garlic clove. Mix the flour and ½ cup of the milk in a small bowl and stir until smooth. Stir this mixture into the simmering broth. Add the rest of the milk. Cook for about 4 minutes, stirring occasionally. Add the broccoli and cook until broccoli is tender, or for about 5 minutes. Lower the heat and while stirring, slowly add the shredded cheese into the soup. Do not let the soup boil after cheese has been added or cheese will separate. Stir in Worcestershire sauce and serve.

Makes 4 servings at 270 calories per serving.

NEW ENGLAND CLAM CHOWDER

12 oz shucked clams, chopped
2 c potatoes, raw, diced
¼ c celery, finely chopped
¼ c carrot, finely chopped
⅓ c chopped onion
2 c lowfat milk
2 tbsp all-purpose flour
2 tsp butter or margarine
1 tsp Worcestershire sauce

Drain clams and reserve liquid. Add enough water to clam juice to measure 1½ cups. Add clam juice to a large saucepan with potatoes, celery, carrots, and onions. Cover and cook for about 15 minutes or until potatoes are tender. Stir in clams and 1½ cups of the milk. Combine remaining ½ cup of milk with the flour and stir into chowder. Add butter. Cook and stir until thickened and bubbly. Stir in Worcestershire sauce.

Makes 4 servings at 305 calories per serving.

DESSERTS AND QUICK BREADS

FRESH STRAWBERRY PIE

4½ c fresh strawberries, cleaned and hulled
1 c strawberry juice or nectar
1 envelope Knox unflavored gelatin
½ c unbleached flour
1½ tbsp margarine or butter
1 tbsp ice water
1 c plain lowfat yogurt
1 tsp vanilla
2 tsp fructose

Cut large strawberries in half. Keep medium and small strawberries whole. Set aside.

Make crust by blending flour, margarine, and water into a dough. Roll out into a 9-inch pan. Bake at 375°F for 10 minutes or until crust is golden brown. Let cool.

Arrange strawberries onto crust. Dissolve gelatin into 1 cup of juice. Cook over low heat until completely dissolved. Cool. Pour slowly and carefully over strawberries. Refrigerate for 2 hours. Garnish pie with yogurt, vanilla, and fructose mixture.

Makes 6 servings at 110 calories per serving.

TROPICAL PINEAPPLE-MERINGUE SLICES

pineapple slices (8 rings, each ½-inch thick)
⅓ c raisins
½ c walnuts, chopped
2 egg whites
2 tsp lemon juice
⅓ c fructose
½ tsp grated lemon rind
2 tbsp coconut, shredded, unsweetened

Place pineapple rings on a large baking sheet. Place under the broiler to lightly brown, carefully watching not to burn. Then fill the cavity of each slice with a mixture of the raisins and walnuts. Beat the egg whites until soft peaks form. Add lemon juice and beat until stiff. Add fructose, 2 tablespoons at a time, beating after each addition. Add lemon rind. Top each pineapple slice with egg white mixture and sprinkle with coconut. Bake in a 350°F oven for 15 minutes or until meringue turns lightly golden brown.

Makes 8 servings at 100 calories per serving.

CITRON ALASKA

4 large oranges, thick skinned
2 c plain lowfat yogurt
1 tsp fructose
2 tbsp frozen orange juice concentrate, defrosted
2 tsp orange-flavored liqueur
1 tsp orange zest
2 egg whites
¼ tsp cream of tartar
2 tbsp fructose
¼ tsp vanilla

Cut 1 inch off of the top of each orange. Using a grapefruit spoon or knife, scoop out the orange pulp; save it for another recipe. Mix the yogurt, fructose, orange juice concentrate, liqueur, and orange zest. Spoon into the orange shells and place in the freezer until firm.

Before serving, beat the egg whites on low speed until foamy. Add the tartar and gradually add the fructose and vanilla, beating on high speed until mixture is stiff and glossy. Spread the meringue over each of the orange shells. Place the oranges on a baking sheet and place in the upper part of a 400°F preheated oven. Bake no more than 4 minutes, long enough for the meringue to turn golden brown. Watch carefully while in the oven.

Garnish with orange or lemon leaves to serve.

Makes 4 servings at 120 calories per serving.

STRAWBERRY MERINGUES

4 egg whites
¾ c fructose
½ tsp cream of tartar
1 tsp vanilla

1 tsp grated orange peel
4 c strawberries, hulled and halved
*8 heaping tbsp Light-Whipped Topping
3 tbsp melted semisweet chocolate chips

Beat egg whites until soft peaks form. Add cream of tartar and vanilla and beat until stiff. Add fructose a little at a time beating after each addition. Add orange peel. To make the meringue shell, drop 2 large tablespoons of egg white mixture on a foil-lined baking sheet. With a spoon, press down on the center to make a depression, forming the shell. Bake at 250°F for 30 to 35 minutes, or until pale golden in color. Then turn off oven and allow meringue shells to dry out in the oven for at least 3 hours. (Another way to form meringue shells is to fill a pastry bag with the egg white mixture and pipe concentric circles, about 3 inches in diameter, and ¾ inch in height.)

To serve, arrange strawberries in the center of the shells, top with 1 tablespoon of Light-Whipped Topping, and drizzle shell with a small amount of melted chocolate.

Makes 8 servings at 100 calories per serving.

---

*See recipe for Light-Whipped Topping.

LIGHT CHOCOLATE CHEESECAKE

16 oz package ricotta cheese, part skim
2 eggs
¼ c fructose
1 tbsp cocoa powder
¼ c plain yogurt
2 tsp vanilla
3 egg whites
¼ tsp cream of tartar
chocolate wafer crumb crust

In a mixing bowl, combine cheese, eggs, fructose, cocoa, yogurt, and vanilla. With an electric mixer, mix at low speed until ingredients are well blended. Increase speed on mixer until ingredients are smooth. In another bowl, beat the egg whites with the cream of tartar until stiff but not dry. Fold the egg white mixture gently into the cheese mixture. Pour into the chocolate wafer crumb crust and bake at 325°F for 35 minutes, or until wood pick inserted into the center comes out clean. Cool on a rack. Chill for 8 hours before serving to allow this delicate cake to set.

Makes 10 servings at 150 calories per serving.

CHOCOLATE WAFER CRUMB CRUST

20 chocolate wafers
1½ tbsp butter

Crush the wafers in a food processor or place wafers between sheets of plastic wrap and crush with a rolling pin. Mix crumbs with the butter and press into a 9-inch spring-form pan.

RASPBERRY SHERBET

2 c milk, lowfat
⅓ c fructose
1 envelope unflavored gelatin
2 c fresh or plain frozen and drained raspberries
 (may use any fruit such as peaches, nectarines, or
 plums)
½ c orange juice
2 tbsp lemon juice

In a saucepan, combine milk, fructose, and gelatin. Stir over low heat until fructose and gelatin are dissolved. Place milk mixture and all remaining ingredients in electric blender and puree. Turn into a metal ice cube tray or a 9 x 5 x 3-inch loaf pan. Freeze until outer edge of mixture is solid but center is still mushy. Pour mixture into a mixing bowl and beat until smooth and fluffy. Return to freezer and freeze until firm.

Makes about 1 quart. Contains 110 calories per ⅔ cup serving.

APRICOT STRUDEL

12 small apricots or 8 med, sliced
1 tbsp cornstarch
8 filo or strudel sheets
¼ c margarine or butter, melted

Place sliced apricots into a bowl. Mix with the cornstarch. On a waxpaper lined wooden board, place

2 filo sheets and brush lightly with margarine or butter. Place 2 more sheets on top and brush with margarine or butter. Continue process until 8 more sheets are used. Carefully wrap filo between the brushings so that it does not dry up. Place apricot mixture on one end of the sheets of filo. Roll like a strudel, tucking sides in and not allowing apricot mixture to leak through the seams. Place on a baking sheet and brush with more margarine or butter. Bake for 25 minutes at 375°F (or until golden brown).

Makes 4 servings at 110 calories per serving.

GLAZED PEACH PIE

3½ c sliced peaches (fresh or canned in juice)
1 tbsp lemon juice
1 c peach juice
1 packet unflavored gelatin (2 tsp)
1–9-inch graham cracker crust

Peel peaches, if using fresh, and slice into ¼-inch slices. Sprinkle with lemon juice. In a small saucepan, add ½ cup of the peach juice and sprinkle the gelatin over the juice to soften it. Bring the mixture to a low simmer until gelatin is completely dissolved. Remove from heat, and stir in remaining peach juice. Arrange 1 layer of peaches over the crust. Slowly drizzle half the peach syrup over the peaches until each peach is covered. Arrange 1 more layer of peaches over this and drizzle remaining peach syrup. Refrigerate until set, or for about 1 hour.

GRAHAM CRACKER CRUST

¾ c plain graham cracker crumbs
1 tbsp butter or margarine
½ tsp cinnamon

Fork-blend crumbs and butter thoroughly. Press mixture into a lightly greased pie plate. Bake in a preheated 400°F oven for 5 minutes. Cool before filling.

Makes 7 servings at 145 calories per serving.

LIGHT BANANA CREAM PIE

1 envelope unflavored gelatin
½ c cold water
¼ c fructose
1½ c plain, lowfat yogurt
1 tsp vanilla
2 small bananas, thinly sliced

CRUST
¾ c plain graham cracker crumbs
1½ tbsp margarine
½ tsp cinnamon

Fork-blend crumbs and margarine thoroughly. Press mixture into a lightly greased pie plate. Bake in a preheated 400°F oven for 5 minutes. Cool.

Combine gelatin and cold water in a saucepan. Bring to a boil to dissolve, stirring carefully. Remove from heat. Mix in yogurt, fructose, and vanilla. Spread half the filling into the pie crust; cover with a layer of banana slices. Then top with remaining filling. Chill until set.

Makes 8 servings at 120 calories per serving.

ORANGE WHEAT GERM CAKE

1 orange, unpeeled, sliced horizontally, very thinly
⅓ c fructose
½ c unbleached flour
½ c whole wheat flour
¼ c toasted wheat germ
1 tsp baking powder
1¼ tsp baking soda
1 egg
1 tbsp oil
1 tsp vanilla
1 tsp grated orange peel
½ c plain yogurt, lowfat
2 tbsp milk

Preheat oven to 350°F. Put the orange slices in a small saucepan to which water has been added to cover slices. Simmer for 10 minutes, then drain. Arrange

slices in the bottom of a nonstick round cake pan. Set
aside. In a small mixing bowl, stir together the fructose,
both flours, wheat germ, and baking powder and baking soda. In another bowl, beat the egg; add the oil,
vanilla, orange peel, yogurt, and milk and mix until
smooth. Gradually stir the dry ingredients into the
liquid ingredients until all are thoroughly moistened.
Pour into the cake pan. Bake at 350°F for about 20
minutes or until wooden pick inserted into the center
comes out clean. Cool cake pan for about 15 minutes,
loosen the sides of the pan with a fork, and reverse cake
onto a serving dish, orange slices up.

Makes 8 servings at 140 calories per serving.

PEAR CAKE

1 c whole wheat flour
⅓ c fructose
1 tsp cinnamon
1½ tbsp butter or margarine
½ tsp baking soda
1 tsp vanilla
¼ c milk
¼ c yogurt, plain
1 egg
3 med pears, peeled, chopped
¼ c walnuts, ground

Combine flour, fructose, and cinnamon. Cut in the
butter with a pastry blender until the mixture is crumbly.
Remove ⅓ cup and set aside. Stir the baking soda into
remaining crumbs. Beat milk, yogurt, vanilla, and egg
and mix into crumb mixture. Blend in pears. Pour into
a lightly greased 9-inch cake pan. Mix the reserved
crumb mixture with the walnuts and sprinkle on top.
Bake in a 375°F oven for about 30 minutes or until a
wooden pick inserted in the center comes out clean.

Makes 10 servings at 130 calories per serving.

KRISTA'S COOKIES

2½ tbsp butter or margarine
1½ tbsp fructose
½ c whole wheat flour

½ tsp baking soda
½ c chopped dried fruit (may use dates, apricots, or raisins)
1 egg
½ tsp vanilla
¼ c chopped nuts (walnuts or pecans)
¼ tsp allspice

Cream butter. Add fructose. Cream until smooth. In small bowl add flour, baking soda, and dried fruit. Mix. Beat egg until fluffy and add to creamed fat. To butter mixture add flour mixture in thirds, stirring after each addition. Toss in nuts and mix lightly. Use teaspoon to drop 24 cookies on a nonstick cookie sheet. Bake at 350°F for 10 minutes or until toothpick inserted in cookie comes out clean.

Makes 24 servings at 41 calories per serving.

CRANBERRY CAKE

1 c whole wheat flour
1 c unbleached all-purpose flour
⅓ c fructose
1½ tsp baking powder
½ tsp baking soda
½ tsp salt (optional)
3 tbsp butter or margarine
1 tbsp grated orange peel
½ c buttermilk
¼ c orange juice
1 egg, well beaten
1 c cranberries, chopped

Spray bottom and sides of round layer cake pan with nonstick spray. Mix flours, fructose, baking powder, baking soda, and salt. Stir in butter until mixture is crumbly. Stir in orange peel, buttermilk, juice, and egg just until flour is moistened. Stir in cranberries. Spread mixture in pan. Bake at 350°F for about 45 minutes or until wooden pick inserted in center comes out clean.

Makes 12 servings at 132 calories per serving.

SPICY STUFFED PEARS

4 ripe pears
4 tbsp raisins or chopped dates

4 tsp walnuts, chopped
¼ tsp cinnamon
¼ tsp ginger

Slice off top of each pear about 1 inch down from
stem, leaving stem on. Set tops aside. Core pears using
an apple corer or a thin bladed knife, being careful not
to cut through bottom of fruit. Mix raisins, walnuts,
and spices together. Stuff each pear with ¼ of this
mixture. Cover with pear tops and set in a baking dish
to which ½ inch of water has been added. Bake for
about 35–40 minutes or until pears are tender. If pears
brown too quickly, cover loosely with foil.

Makes 4 servings at 100 calories per serving.

STRIPED FRUIT GEL

4 tsp unflavored gelatin powder
¾ c raspberries
¾ c unsweetened raspberry juice or puree, or red
   grape juice
½ c pineapple juice, canned
¼ c crushed pineapple, canned
¾ c plain lowfat yogurt
¾ c blueberries
¾ c unsweetened blueberry juice or puree, or red
   grape juice

In a small saucepan, soften 1 heaping measuring
teaspoon of gelatin in ¼ cup of the raspberry juice. Stir
constantly over medium heat until all the gelatin is
dissolved. Remove from heat. Stir in remaining raspberry juice and gently stir in raspberries. Pour into a
2-quart capacity mold. Refrigerate until it gels, for
about 30 minutes.

In a small saucepan, soften 1 heaping measuring
teaspoon of gelatin in ¼ cup of the pineapple juice.
Stir constantly over medium heat until all the gelatin is
dissolved. Remove from heat. Stir in remaining pineapple juice, pineapple, and yogurt. Pour over raspberry
layer when raspberry layer has gelled.

In a small saucepan soften 1 heaping measuring
teaspoon of gelatin in ¼ cup of the blueberry juice. Stir
constantly over medium heat until all the gelatin is

dissolved. Remove from heat. Stir in remaining juice and blueberries. Pour over pineapple-yogurt layer when that layer has gelled.

Makes 6 servings at 85 calories per serving.

CALIFORNIA FRUIT TORTE

1 envelope unflavored gelatin
10 small grapes, seedless
1 c strawberries
½ c canned pineapple slices, packed in juice
2 canned peach halves, packed in juice

Combine peach and pineapple juices, and set aside 2 cups. Cut peach halves into 6 pieces. Halve the strawberries and pineapple. Arrange fruit on a 9-inch glass pie plate, making concentric circles of the various fruit.

Take ½ cup of the fruit juice and combine with gelatin in a saucepan over medium heat until completely dissolved. Stir in remaining 1½ cups of fruit juice. Chill mixture until it is the consistency of unbeaten egg whites. Carefully pour half of the chilled gelatin mixture over the fruit and chill in the refrigerator until set. Then add the remaining gelatin mixture and chill "torte" until set. Cut torte into 6 wedges.

Makes 6 servings at 65 calories per serving.

OATMEAL MUFFINS

1⅓ c whole wheat flour
⅔ c oats
3 tsp baking powder
¼ tsp salt (optional)
3 tbsp fructose
¼ tsp cinnamon
¼ tsp ginger
1 egg
1 c milk
2 tbsp oil
⅔ c raisins or currants

Combine flour, oats, baking powder, salt, fructose, cinnamon, and ginger. Beat the egg with the milk and oil in a small bowl. Stir into dry ingredients along with raisins. Mix only enough to moisten all ingredients.

Spoon into 12 nonstick muffin cups and bake in a 375°F oven for about 20 minutes or until lightly browned.

Makes 12 servings at 122 calories per serving.

PEANUT BUTTER BREAD

⅔ c peanut butter, unsalted with no added oil
3 tbsp fructose
1 egg
1 c unbleached white flour
1 c whole wheat flour
4 tsp baking powder
½ tsp salt (optional)
1 c lowfat milk

Cream peanut butter and fructose. Add egg and beat until mixture is smooth. Add sifted dry ingredients alternately with milk. Beat well and pour onto a greased loaf pan. Bake at 350°F for 50 minutes.

Makes 20 servings at 105 calories per serving.

APPLE OATMEAL COOKIES

½ c unbleached flour
½ c whole wheat flour
½ c fructose
1 tsp baking powder
1 tsp baking soda
¼ tsp cinnamon
¼ c butter
2 eggs
¼ c water
¼ c plain lowfat yogurt
2 c quick-cooking rolled oats
¾ c dried apples, chopped

In a mixing bowl, stir together both flours, fructose, baking soda, baking powder, and cinnamon. Add butter, eggs, water, and yogurt and mix well. Stir in oats and apples. Drop by teaspoonfuls onto a nonstick baking sheet. Bake at 375°F for 8 to 10 minutes.

Makes 6 dozen cookies at 30 calories per cookie.

DRIED APPLES (these taste better than the ones you buy in the store)

Slice 4 apples crosswise, ¼-inch thick. Remove the

core. Place on a nonstick baking sheet and bake at 300°F for about 7 minutes, decreasing the temperature to 200°F for an additional 10 minutes. Remove from oven and chop coarsely.

BROWN RICE AND RAISIN PUDDING

1 c long grain brown rice
1 c water
3 c milk
1 bay leaf
1 cinnamon stick
1 orange rind
¼ c raisins
1 tsp vanilla
4 tsp fructose

Add rice and bay leaf to boiling water. Cover and simmer for 15 minutes. Add 2 cups of milk. Partly cover and simmer for 10 minutes or until rice is tender. Add the rest of the milk, cinnamon stick, orange rind, and raisins. Cook over low heat until thickened, stirring occasionally. Stir in vanilla and fructose. May be served hot or cold.

Makes 6⅔ cup servings at 145 calories per serving.

CHOCOLATE MOUSSE

2 c lowfat milk
1 pkg (.25 oz) unflavored gelatin
2 tsp cocoa powder
2 tsp fructose
1 tsp vanilla
3 egg whites

Dissolve gelatin in ¼ cup of the milk. Add cocoa powder and fructose. Gently heat mixture until gelatin and cocoa dissolve. Add this mixture to remaining milk. Stir in vanilla. Pour into a bowl and refrigerate until mixture has the consistency of a milkshake.

Meanwhile beat the 3 egg whites until stiff peaks form. Carefully blend into thickened milk mixture. Pour into 4 parfait glasses. Refrigerate until firm.

Makes 4 servings at 90 calories per serving.

FLAN (CARAMEL CUSTARD)

½ c fructose
¼ c water
1 stick cinnamon
3 eggs
1 tsp vanilla extract
2½ c lowfat milk, scalded
1 tsp grated orange peel (optional)

In a small saucepan, add the water, ¼ cup of the fructose, and the cinnamon stick. Bring to a boil, gently shaking the pan to dissolve the fructose. Boil over a low heat until it turns golden brown, for about 15 to 20 minutes. Pour into a 1-quart, round baking dish or mold and swirl to coat the syrup onto the sides. Then beat the eggs in a small bowl, adding the remaining fructose and vanilla. Slowly stir in the cooled, scalded milk. Stir in the orange peel. Pour into the baking dish or mold. Place dish in a larger baking pan to which water has been added to come halfway up the sides of the baking dish. Bake in a 300°F oven for about 45 minutes or until a wooden pick inserted in the center comes out clean. Remove dish from the water and allow to cool before refrigerating. Before serving, immerse dish into hot water for about 20 seconds and invert onto a serving dish.

Makes 6 servings at 155 calories per serving.

SWEET CHEESE CREPES

1 c + 2 tbsp unbleached flour
1 c + 2 tbsp lowfat milk
2 eggs
1 tsp oil
1 tsp butter or margarine

In a blender or with a mixer combine the flour, milk, eggs, and oil. Beat until well blended and smooth. Chill batter for about 30 minutes.

Lightly grease a 6-inch nonstick skillet or crepe pan with a little of the butter and place over medium heat until pan is hot. Remove pan from heat and spoon in about 2 tablespoons of the batter. Rotate and tilt the skillet to spread the batter evenly over the pan bottom. Return the pan to medium heat and cook the crepe until lightly browned on the edges. Flip crepe and cook underside for about 1 minute. Place cooked crepes on a paper towel. Repeat process until all crepes are cooked. Wipe skillet with a small amount of butter between crepes. Crepes may be stacked between sheets of plastic wrap and frozen.

Makes about 15 servings at 50 calories per serving.

SWEET CHEESE FILLING

3 tbsp golden raisins
¾ c lowfat cottage cheese
¼ c frozen orange juice concentrate
1 tsp grated orange peel
½ tsp vanilla
dash of nutmeg and ground cloves

Plump raisins by soaking in ¼ cup of hot water. Let stand for 15 minutes. Drain water. Combine all ingredients. Spoon 2 tablespoons of filling onto each crepe. Fold crepe in quarters. Warm filled crepe thoroughly on a warm skillet. Serve at once.

Fills 8 crepes at 95 calories per filled crepe.

SWEET POTATO PIE

2 lbs cooked sweet potatoes
2 tbsp fructose
2 eggs, slightly beaten
1½ c lowfat milk
1 tbsp orange juice
½ tsp cinnamon
½ tsp ginger
¼ tsp nutmeg
1 tsp grated orange peel
"light" topping

Mash sweet potatoes or puree in a blender. You should have 2 cups of potatoes. Add fructose and eggs. Mix well. Gradually stir in milk and all other ingredients. Pour into a 9-inch pie pan. Bake for about 45 minutes at 350°F or until knife inserted in middle comes out clean. May top each serving with "light" topping.

Makes 8 servings at 135 calories per serving.

"LIGHT" TOPPING

1 tsp unflavored gelatin
¼ c cold water
3 tsp fructose
1 tsp vanilla
¼ c whipping cream
4 eggs at room temperature
½ tsp cream of tartar

Stir gelatin in ¼ cup of cold water in a small saucepan. Over medium heat, stir until gelatin dissolves. Pour into a small bowl, stirring in fructose, vanilla, and cream. Refrigerate until set, for about 1 hour.

Meanwhile, dip whole eggs into boiling water that has been removed from the heat. Submerge eggs for 30 seconds. Remove and separate whites from eggs. Beat until foamy; add cream of tartar; then continue beating until stiff. Beat gelatin mixture until creamy; then fold into egg whites. Refrigerate until ready to use. Best used within 1 hour.

Makes about 2½ cups at 7 calories per tablespoon.

BEVERAGES

LOW CALORIE COOL DRINKS

1. Orange Soda
   2 tbsp frozen orange juice concentrate, unsweetened
   8 oz club soda or carbonated water
   Stir together. Add ice cubes.
   50 calories per 8-ounce serving

2. Grape Soda
   2 tbsp frozen grape juice concentrate, unsweetened
   8 oz club soda or carbonated water
   Stir together. Add ice cubes.
   50 calories per 8-ounce serving

3. Melon Frappé
   ¼ med cantaloupe, chilled, cut in pieces
   8 oz lowfat milk
   Mix in blender for about 1 minute.
   190 calories per 12-ounce serving

4. Strawberry Milkshake
   ¾ c fresh strawberries, chilled
   1 c lowfat milk
   ½ tsp vanilla
       Mix in blender for 1 minute.
       190 calories per 12-ounce serving

5. Fruit Punch
   1 tbsp frozen concentrated pineapple juice,
       unsweetened
   1 tbsp frozen concentrated orange juice, unsweetened
   twist of lemon
   8 oz club soda or carbonated water
       Stir together. Add ice cubes.
       50 calories per 8-ounce serving

8 / How to Reduce the Calories of Your Favorite Recipes

The recipes on the preceding pages will help you in your daily menu selection. However, you may want to convert some of your favorite recipes into lower calorie versions. There are several ways in which the calories in a recipe can be reduced. First, the method of cooking the food or constituent foods in the recipe can be modified to decrease the total calorie content. For instance, when a recipe calls for frying, you may be able to "fry" with little or no added fat, or you may "oven" fry. Second, the foods called for in a recipe may be substituted for lower calorie products. For example, lowfat milk can replace cream in most dishes. Lastly, the quantity of a particular food in a recipe may be reduced. For example, when baking cookies, the fat can easily be cut by ½ to ⅔ without sacrificing taste, although the texture will usually be slightly less crisply. Also, the sugar content of the cookie can be cut by ½ to ⅔, or fructose may be used to reduce the quantity of sweetness needed.

Listed here are commonly used methods of food preparation and suitable substitutions.

Frying: You will probably want to invest in a few nonstick skillets. Most foods will brown nicely over a medium flame without the addition of any fat. Lean ground meat and chicken pieces will brown if not too crowded in the pan. Pancakes, French toast, and potatoes will also brown nicely. You may also use a well-seasoned iron pan for "frying." An iron skillet will last a lifetime and you don't have to worry about scratching it. To "cure" an iron skillet, scrub your new or old iron pan thoroughly. Put a tablespoon or so of oil in it and spread it around to completely cover the surface of the pan. Place the pan on moderate heat until the oil starts to smoke. Then turn the heat off and cool the pan. When the pan cools, wipe off all the oil with a paper towel. Repeat this process one more time and your pan will be "cured." Do not wash a "cured" pan with water. When you have finished cooking in it, wipe it and it's ready to be used again. You may need to rub off with salt anything that has stuck on the pan. Wiping the bottom of the pan with about ½ teaspoon of oil before each use will keep your pan "cured." You may need to recure your iron skillet several times a year, depending on how frequently you use it.

Another low calorie frying substitute is oven "frying." Chicken and fish are especially tasty this way. Recipes for each are found in the preceding chapter. Vegetables such as eggplant slices and zucchini sticks or sliced potatoes may also be oven "fried" with little or no fat. Just use a nonstick baking sheet without fat. If you choose to use some fat, brush a little oil on the food before baking.

Sautéing: You may sauté meats or vegetables in a nonstick skillet with a little water or in their own juices. No need to add any fat at all.

The following is a listing of common ingredients which are high in calories and which may be substituted with a lower calorie product:

SUBSTITUTION LIST

HIGH CALORIE	LOWER CALORIE
Fats (oils, butter, and margarine)	Omit entirely or, if baking, reduce by ½ to ⅓. Enhance flavor of food by adding more herbs and spices.
Cream, whipped cream	Use lowfat milk. Use "light cream topping" for whipped cream (recipe in chapter 7).
Sugar, honey	Reduce the quantity by ½ to ⅔. Fructose may be substituted for sugar. Use 1 part fructose to substitute for 2 parts sugar.
Chocolate	Use cocoa powder which is very low in fat, or carob powder, found in health food stores.
Sour cream	Use plain lowfat yogurt or use a blended mixture of lowfat cottage cheese with lowfat yogurt.
Sausage and bacon	Omit or use lean ground pork with sausage seasonings.
Mayonnaise	Use plain lowfat yogurt or a mixture of small parts of mayonnaise with yogurt. Commercial low calorie mayonnaise has ½ the calories of regular mayonnaise.
Cheeses	Use lowfat mozarella, lowfat cottage cheese, lowfat ricotta cheese, or any cheese with less than 20% fat.
Jam, jelly, preserves	Use sugar-reduced jams.
Beef, high fat cuts	Use round, flank, shank cuts such as London broil or sir-

SUBSTITUTION LIST

	loin. Use hamburger which contains less than 20% fat, or grind your own from the above cuts.
Flavored gelatin	Use unflavored gelatin and unsweetened fruit juices. One packet. (.25 oz) will gel 2 c liquid.

You can see from the recipes in chapter 7 that most of these substitutions were made in those recipes. You will need to experiment a bit to find the proper quantities and combinations for the lower calorie version of your favorite recipe. Certain items, such as rich pastries and desserts are simply not convertible as they rely too much on fat and sugar for their taste. Less calorically dense and equally delicious desserts can be created using fruits, fresh or dried, as a basis, or using a combination of fruits and starches and/or milk products. Lower-caloried fruit pies and tarts are good examples of desserts which can be converted. Similarly, recipes for puddings, custards, gelatins, and mousses can be adjusted to reduce the calories by substituting lower-caloried items as are listed on the substitution list on the previous pages. In most cases, in these desserts, you will be reducing fat and sugar content.

For many recipes, you will be able to calculate the number of food units per serving portion, and from this, you can calculate the calorie content. Using a combination entrée dish as an example:

SPANISH RICE CASSEROLE—Serves 4

	1 portion yields:
2 c cooked rice	½ c rice = 1 starch unit
¾ c chopped celery	vegetables as desired
¼ c chopped green pepper	vegetables as desired
1 med onion, chopped	vegetables as desired

1 c chopped tomatoes in puree	vegetables as desired
¾ lb lean ground beef	$\dfrac{12 \text{ oz}}{4} = 3$ oz *raw* ground beef = 2¼ oz = about 2 meat units

From this recipe, you can see that one serving, ¼, of the Spanish rice casserole is equal to 1 starch unit, 2 meat, and 2 vegetable units, which can be used freely. This example was fairly easy; you might find recipes which do not break down into such neat unit sizes. For instance, if the recipe called for 3 cups of cooked rice, 3 cups divided by 4 servings is ¾ of a cup per person. Half a cup of rice is 1 starch unit; therefore, ¾ of a cup is 1½ starch units. Similarly, the recipe could have called for more meat in which case 1 portion would be greater than 2 meat units. Develop the habit of breaking down a recipe to calculate the food units it contains, from which you can also extrapolate the calorie content. Referring back to the same casserole, we calculated that it contains

	Calories
1 starch unit	70
2 meat units	130
⅝ c vegetables	30
Total Calories	238

The average calorie value of common foods is given with the food unit lists in chapter 6. The original recipe for the Spanish rice casserole called for 2 tablespoons of butter in which to sauté the vegetables, but this process is totally unnecessary and saves 270 calories in the entire recipe or about 67 calories per serving (270 total calories/4 servings = 67).

The same basic method of calculation can be used to determine the calorie value and food units of any recipe. However, in the case of a more complex recipe, especially a recipe for a baked good such as muffins or cookies, the calculation takes longer. For that, you will require a more detailed list of the calorie levels of foods, such as in the book *Food Values of Portions Commonly*

Used by Bowes and Church. For the most part you will probably be using entrée recipes on your daily menu, and not desserts. Detailed calculations for the calorie value of your recipes will not be necessary, especially if you use chapter 7 as a guide.

9 / The Trials of Daily Living

Throughout the course of the day, you will be involved in situations in which your actions impact on your ability to comply with your diet plan, and on your ability to lose weight. These situations include meal planning, grocery selection, eating away from home, holiday and party eating, and lunch packing, among others. In this chapter each of these issues will be discussed as well as the special dietary needs during pregnancy, adaptation of the Alive and Well Diet for vegetarians, and the high iron requirements of women of child-bearing age.

Meal Planning

As much as possible, take some time to plan a basic weekly menu. This way you will be sure that your meals are thought out in terms of calories, nutrients, and expenses. You may use the menus in chapter 7 as a guide. If you are working outside the home, or for any reason are unable to spend much time in meal preparation, select menus and recipes which are the easiest to prepare. Dinner and lunch meals require more plan-

175

ning than breakfast. Starting with the protein foods first, on a seven-day menu plan, you can include chicken for at least two dinners and some lunches, beef for about two dinners or lunches, fish, depending on its availability, as often as you like, with turkey, lean pork and lamb for variety. Use legumes such as kidney beans, dry peas, and white beans as meat substitutes for dinner or lunch once or twice a week. Remember that ½ cup of cooked beans is equivalent in calories and protein to 1 starch unit plus 1 meat unit. So 1 cup of cooked split green peas is the same as having 2 ounces of meat and 2 slices of bread. Alternate the starches at your meals from among potatoes, rice, pasta, or bread, to name a few. Each dinner or lunch should include 1 or more vegetables. At dinner, include 1 steamed vegetable and a fresh salad. Fruit will most often form the basis of your dessert. The recipes in chapter 7 will give you a chance to create fancy but nutritious and low calorie desserts such as gels, pies, and some cakes.

If you, like so many of us, have just about 30 minutes to prepare dinner from start to finish, do a little preplanning. Make sure you take the chicken or meat out of the freezer the night before and let it thaw out in the refrigerator. If you are planning to cook dry beans, be sure to sort and soak them the night before. A pressure cooker will allow you to make soups and stews and many dishes in a fraction of the time. A microwave oven, much costlier, also reduces the cooking time. Food does not have to be complicated to be good.

Shopping for Food

By controlling the food that enters your home, you can gain better control over what you eat, which impacts on your weight loss. If a high calorie, low nutrient food is sitting in your cupboard, tempting you, you might finally eat it. If you had never purchased that food item, you would not have the opportunity to eat it. That is the point. You must readjust your way of shopping to create opportunities which will positively, not negatively, impact on your diet. First, do not do your grocery shopping on an empty stomach. Always do your shopping after you have eaten. Studies have shown that you will probably purchase more food when you are hungry. It has been demonstrated that overweight people overreact to the visual and sensory cues associated with food and eating as compared to leaner people. For instance, in the overweight, hunger is signaled more by external factors such as pictures of foods, descriptions of food, and the hour of the day than by actual physiological hunger. Being bombarded in the supermarket by advertisements of delicious food is of no help to the person who wants to stay with a diet. The temptations are even greater if you are hungry. The moral of this is to shop after your meals, on a full and satisfied stomach. Rule number two is, shop only from your grocery list. Your grocery list should reflect what you need to purchase for your meals in the coming days, or if you shop weekly, for the week. Plan your meals in advance, and make your shopping list accordingly. You may want to keep a running shopping list in your kitchen. On this running list, you write down those items, as you think of them, that you will need to purchase next time at the supermarket. When you realize that you have used the last drop of the wine vinegar, jot that down on a list. By having a complete, planned shopping list, you will have some "support" as you shop by the numerous temptations. After all, if you can avoid bringing into the house the problem-causing foods in the first place, you will not have to battle with the temptations later. Do not make purchase decisions in the supermarket. Rather, follow your shopping list very carefully.

One other rule, and this one is one that, if you are carefully following the Alive and Well Diet, will be automatic, is to buy foods that are as unprocessed as possible, and which require some preparation prior to consumption. Any food that can be eaten immediately should be avoided. When food takes some preparation before it can be consumed, you will have some time to think about your eating. Your perception of hunger can change quickly. If you feel hunger but become distracted by another activity, you may find that your hunger has dissipated. By involving yourself in the preparation of what you are going to eat, you are increasing the amount of time between your impulse to eat and actual eating. In this time interval you will have a chance to control or channel the impulse to eat.

Let's turn to what actually should go on your shopping list. First, your shopping list can be organized into several groups which will help you with your meal planning, and reduce your time in the supermarket by making your shopping more efficient. Organize your shopping list into the following categories: meat, produce, dairy, bakery, staple dry goods, frozen foods, and condiments. If you shop weekly you will be able to check your weekly planned menus against this list. Supermarkets are organized into sections similar to the organization of your list so you will only have to go down an aisle once.

Within the meat group, depending on your weekly menu, an item that you will probably want to include on your list is chicken, preferably chicken breasts. Because chicken is so versatile, you can include it in at least two meals during the week. Other good selections are turkey breasts, which you can divide in half to be frozen for future use, round or flank steak, lean pork or lamb chops, or roasts such as round roast. When you purchase large pieces of meat, cut them into pieces that you or your family can eat in one meal. Wrap each piece individually before freezing. If you are cooking just for yourself, cut the meat into individual 4-ounce raw weight pieces and freeze so that you can take just one portion out as needed. Meat and chicken usually lose 25 percent of their weight from cooking. Therefore, 4 ounces raw becomes 3 ounces cooked weight. Three ounces raw weight becomes about 2¼ ounces cooked. Fresh or plain frozen fish are items you can include on your list. Do not use breaded fish sticks or patties.

In the produce section, you can select seasonal fruits and vegetables. Standard vegetables which are available almost all season long are carrots and celery, various kinds of lettuce, tomatoes, green peppers, onions, and cabbage. Various squash, green beans, broccoli, and spinach are usually plentiful and lend themselves to a variety of cooking methods. If the produce selection is poor or if certain items are unavailable you can purchase plain frozen vegetables. Do not buy vegetables with sauces or added butter as these are higher in calories. You can keep a few potatoes in your pantry or refrigerator and use them throughout the week. Be sure to explore and experiment with vegetables and fruits with which you may not be familiar. Variety in taste, texture, and color make your meals more interesting and variety assures you of getting a number of different nutrients. Fresh fruits can be one of the most delightful parts of your meal. With the money that you are saving by not buying prepared pastry, convenience foods, and the like, you will be able to splurge with the most beautiful, fragrant fruit you can find. Try various berries, tropical fruit, and the pick of the crop of seasonal fruits for dessert. When certain fruits are out of season, you may purchase canned fruits. Select only canned fruits which are packed in juice or water. Even fruit packed in light syrup has too much sugar. Frozen fruit is also available. Again, do not buy fruit packed with sugar. Read the label carefully and it should read only fruit, no sugar or corn syrup.

In the dairy section, select fresh lowfat milk, or nonfat milk which, because it contains no fat, is even lower in calories. There are many things that you can do with plain lowfat yogurt. You can use it as a dressing or topping and in sauces. Yogurt may earn a permanent place on your shopping list. Your list may include lowfat cottage cheese, hoop cheese, lowfat mozarella, and any other lowfat cheese you may find. Unfortunately, there are not very many lowfat cheeses available. The processed cheese slices which are advertised as being lowfat are indeed lowfat. However, to me, they lack in taste, and are very high in sodium. Feta, a flavorful Greek cheese, is relatively low in fat, but high in sodium. Another lowfat cheese is sapsago from Switzerland. It is good but expensive. In small quantities, you can use a sharp grated cheese such as Parmesan for flavor. On the Alive and Well Diet you have the choice of using butter or margarine. The Alive and Well Diet is low in total fat content, comprising about 30 percent of the total calories. Of that fat, nearly equal proportions should come from saturated fat and polyunsaturated and monosaturated fats. By including vegetable oils, meat, dairy products, vegetables, and grains in your diet, you will have a mix of various fats. If you like margarine, you may use this. I personally prefer the taste of real butter.

In the bakery area, you can select from among a variety of whole grain breads. All brown breads are not whole grain, although all whole grains are brownish in color. Often molasses will be added to give flavor and color to a bread which is made of refined flour. Look at the label. Whole wheat flour should be the first ingredient. You can select from sliced bread, rolls, pita bread, and airy or heavy texture breads. Rye and pumpernickle breads are good alternates. There is nothing wrong with refined flour products such as sourdough or French bread. However, do try to include in your daily menu some whole grain products which are higher in fiber and in some nutrients. Calorically, whole grain breads and refined flour breads are very similar. Commercially prepared muffins, biscuits, and croissants are too high in fat. Make your own instead, without the fat, or use a fraction of the fat the recipe calls for.

In the staples group, you should have on hand a variety of goods, which you can use as your "emergency cupboard." More on this later on in this chapter. Items that you can store in your pantry are canned goods, grain foods, and dried foods. We have already discussed some canned fruits you may select. A few cans of plain vegetables are good to have in your pantry for those days when you are out of fresh or frozen vegetables and are unable to shop right away. Canned tomato products such as tomato puree, tomato sauce, and whole tomatoes are good for sauces. Canned kidney beans and garbanzo beans are convenient when you are in a great hurry to prepare a meal. Among the grains, keep brown rice, pasta products, and whole wheat flours available. There are a variety of pastas from which to select. I have found whole wheat, corn, and mixed grain noodles and spaghetti only in large health food stores. Maybe soon they will be available in the supermarkets. Of course you may use regular pasta products, but do not limit yourself to just these. If you like pancakes, there are whole grain pancake mixes available which do not contain added fat. Look for these in your supermarket. Do not select a product which has fat, oil, or lard listed as ingredients. Cereals which have little or no added sugar are the ones you should select. Most brands of cornflakes are not too high in added sugar. Neither are wheat flakes, Grape Nuts, and shredded wheat. Read the label to see if sugar is one of the first ingredients on the label. If so, leave it. Generally, if a product tastes sweet to you, it has too much added sugar. Granola type cereals are loaded with sugar and fat. Cereals which need cooking such as oatmeal and whole wheat cereals should be purchased as plain as possible. Individually packaged instant oatmeal cereals are usually presweetened, and have oil and salt added. Read the label! Another good staple to have on hand is nonfat dry milk powder and evaporated skim or lowfat milk. Both have a long shelf life.

Among frozen foods, the most common ones which you will use are plain frozen vegetables, frozen unsweetened fruits, and fruit juices. There is a wide variety of prepared frozen foods, from pizza to soup. Take the time to make your own, and freeze ahead if you want. There are "diet" frozen dinners, with lower calorie entrées. These are not inexpensive. Some of the products *are* low in calories as a result of being low in fat; however they are usually high in sodium. If you want to be sure that what you are eating is high quality food consistent with your diet plan, make something simple, but make it yourself. If you want a good selection of breads on your daily menus, buy various kinds and freeze them. Take out only what you need and freeze the rest.

Condiments will enhance all the good food that you are already buying. Spices and herbs may be purchased dry and kept for a long time. Fresh herbs are even better when available. Experimentation and preference are your guide. Good vinegars will brighten up your salads. Try herbed vinegars, wine vinegars, and rice vinegars. Oils from which you may select are corn oil, safflower, soybean, sunflower, cottonseed, and olive oil. For flavoring certain dishes you may also use peanut oil or sesame oil, but since you will be using such small amounts, they may not be necessary. Stay away from all food items that contain palm oil or coconut oil as these are very highly saturated fats. They are used largely in the commercial production of foods such as baked goods, cake mixes, and imitation whipped toppings. They are relatively inexpensive fats, and therefore frequently used by the food industry. But since the foods which contain these oils are not part of the Alive and Well Diet, you will probably not be exposed to them.

Prepared mustards, especially the Dijon type, are versatile and low in calories. Sauces such as steak sauces, Worcestershire sauce, and even catsup do contain some sugar and salt, but if used sparingly and occasionally do not contribute a significant amount of calories. They are usually very low in fat content. Soy sauce is very high in sodium. Look for the milder sodium-reduced soy sauce available in large supermarkets that have an Oriental food section. Sugar-reduced jams are now sold next to the regular jams and jellies. You may want to try the various herbal teas available on the store shelves. After a good meal, a good cup of tea, from orange to almond to mint flavored, can be most satisfying and a great final touch.

Eating Out

Eating away from home can present a real test to the dieter. If you are eating in a restaurant with friends who are not themselves following a weight-reducing program, it may be difficult to sit back and watch them indulge in very tempting foods. You will be exposed to many temptations in a restaurant and it is difficult for most of us to resist. Frequently we do not resist. You will have greater "control" if your exposure to visual and sensory cues to eat are limited. So while I am not suggesting that you sit home and pass up dinner invitations, you need to be aware of the risks you are taking. However, you can select a reasonable meal and stay within your diet plan. You should order relatively plainly prepared foods. Start out with a green salad and ask the waiter to hold the dressing or to put it in a cup on the side. Limit yourself to 1 tablespoon of salad dressing. You can dilute the dressing and make it go farther by adding vinegar or lemon juice. You can order club soda or iced tea or tomato juice to drink. If you want to have a drink with the others in your company, limit yourself to one small glass of dry wine. One 3-ounce glass of dry wine contains about 70 calories. Since there are also 70 calories in one starch unit, the wine could be substituted for one of the starch units at that meal. The following list gives the calorie value of common alcoholic beverages:

ALCOHOLIC BEVERAGE	AMOUNT	CALORIES
Distilled spirits		
Gin, vodka, whiskey, or brandy	1 oz	70
Liqueurs	1 oz	60–120
Wines		
Dry, white	3 oz	70
Dry, red	3 oz	60
Champagne, dry	3 oz	90
Beer	6 oz	75

Difficult to pass up is the basket of warm bread with lots of butter which is usually placed on the table even before you place your order. (I told you that restaurants are full of temptations.) If you limit yourself to one slice of bread, you will be within your diet range assuming that you are following the 1,500-calorie plan. You have a choice of whether you want a pat of butter on your bread, dressing on your salad, or a pat of butter on your potato. You may have two fats at this meal so make your choice and stick to it. As far as the entrée is concerned, it is best to order broiled or baked chicken, and remove the skin before you eat it. Avoid sauces and gravies as these are generally too high in fat and therefore too high in calories. Broiled or plain baked fish is another excellent choice. Restaurant portions are usually larger than the portions planned on your diet. The chicken or fish will probably weigh 5 or 6 ounces instead of the 3 ounces allowed on your 1,500-calorie diet plan. Plan ahead and decrease your lunch meal accordingly if you are going out for dinner, or decrease dinner, if you are going out for lunch. Do not skip a meal entirely prior to eating out as chances are that you will be so famished that you will be prone to overeat. The reason why ordering beef, such as a steak or roast, is not recommended is that restaurant cuts are usually more fatty than the round or flank steaks you have been eating on your diet. Also, the portions are too big. For both of these reasons you will consume fewer calories if you select chicken or fish.

For the starch part of your meal, a simple baked potato is your best bet. Most rice pilafs and potato side dishes are prepared with fat. As much as 1 tablespoon of fat can be hidden in that glistening pilaf. Since 1 glass of white wine, about 3 ounces, has 70 calories and because you are allowed 2 starch units for dinner on the 1,500-calorie plan, you could have either the slice of bread and the wine, or the slice of bread and the small baked potato, or the wine and the potato—not all 3. Steamed vegetables are an excellent accompaniment to your meal, but these too usually have added butter or margarine. Explain to your waiter that you cannot have fat such as butter or margarine or oil in your diet due to a medical condition. Explain clearly what you want and if you do so you need not accept anything that is not brought to you the way that you ordered. If you desire soup, select a vegetable soup which is clear, not creamed, or a bouillon. If the soup contains some pasta, figure it into your diet also. For dessert, fresh fruit in season is available almost everywhere. Refer to the table of caloric values of desserts at the end of this section if you have any doubt that fresh cold melon for dessert isn't superior to a brownie à la mode.

When you are invited to eat at a friend's or relative's home you may feel pressure to overeat. Usually the host or hostess has spent some time in preparing good food for their guests. After all this effort and considering that the host's pride is involved, you may fear hurting his feelings if you do not enthusiastically indulge in seconds and desserts. Given your continual efforts to refuse the encouragements from the hosts to take more food, it might seem simpler just to accept the food and eat. Try being candid and honest with your hosts. Tell them that although the food is delicious, that they would be most helpful in letting you stay with your diet by allowing you to help yourself to that which you are able to eat. You have to be firm, but polite at the onset. It would be ideal if you could know the menu before going to the dinner. If you know the hosts well, you can call and ask them, and tell them that you are on a special diet. That way you could preplan what you will eat. You can figure the quantities that you will eat from various foods and stay within your diet. You can calculate the calories of certain desserts you may wish to have in lieu of other foods you would normally have at that meal. For instance, if you want to have a piece of the host's cheesecake and you find that a piece 2" x 2" x 3" has about 200 calories, you would have to omit 200 calories from somewhere else in order to stay within your daily allotted calorie level. You might choose to omit 2 starch units at 140 calories, total, 1 fruit unit at 50 calories to make a grand total of 190 calories saved. You decide what you want to have and in what manner you will modify your diet to accommodate these changes. It is not recommended that you modify your diet frequently to accommodate pastry, desserts, and alcoholic beverages as these foods are nutrient poor. However, occasionally you can make these adjustments which will keep you on your diet and keep you from feeling deprived.

The following list is provided to demonstrate to you the calorie value of some common desserts, and to allow you to *occasionally* make allowances for them in your diet:

CALORIE VALUE FOR DESSERTS

DESSERT	CALORIES
Brownie (2" x 2" x 3¼")	150
Cake	
Angel (¹⁄₁₀ of cake)	120
Chocolate with icing (2" x 2" x 3")	205
Pound (3" x 3" x ½")	140
Cheesecake (2" x 2" x 3")	200
Cookies	
Chocolate chip (3" diam.)	125
Oatmeal (3" diam.)	100
Doughnut	200
Ice cream	
Vanilla (½ c)	145

CALORIE VALUE FOR DESSERTS

DESSERT	CALORIES
Pie	
Fruit (⅙ of 9"-pie)	420
Custard (⅙ of 9"-pie)	365
Sherbet (½ c)	120
Sugar	
Table sugar (1 tsp)	16
Fructose (1 tsp)	16
Honey (1 tsp)	21

Holidays and Parties

The same approach to eating out applies to going to parties or holiday eating. You can make adjustments to your meal plan to keep you within your total calorie quota. Try to plan in advance what you are going to eat, and stick with your plan. If you cannot know beforehand what food will be served, at least find out as soon as you can upon arriving so that you can have time to preplan. This doesn't take the joy away from partying. It's one approach to keep you in control of your eating. With preplanning you avoid the feeling that you have strayed far from your diet, or that you have binged. While we are on the subject, obliterate from your mind entirely the notion that when you have not followed your diet completely you have spoiled everything and all is lost. Don't tell yourself that since you've strayed, you might as well forget the whole thing. If you do, you'll probably return to your old eating patterns. Some flexibility on your diet is allowed on holidays and on very special events. Planning is the key. Knowing the approximate calorie value of the food group units, of alcoholic beverages, of certain desserts, and knowing something about cooking methods, you will probably be able to select foods in appropriate quantities that will be within your diet plan. Hopefully not everything will be deep fat fried or smothered in rich sauces. There almost always are vegetables, cheese, some plain bread, or crackers and club soda. No one at the party will have to know that you are on a diet when you are eating carefully and slowly from what is available.

Eat something before arriving at the party. Do not arrive anywhere on an empty stomach. Do not skip the previous meal so that you'll have extra calories to spend. You will be so hungry by the time the food arrives that you might overeat. If the party meal is at dinner, you can have a lighter lunch, but do not skip it entirely. If the meal is in the middle of the afternoon, have a light lunch, eat wisely at the party, and plan to have a light snack in the evening. Do not carry your food intake account from one day into the next day. If you have gone a little bit over your diet today, do not plan to curtail your food intake even more tomorrow. Food accounts can be only kept for one day. Plan to exercise more instead.

Your spouse or friend can help provide you with support at the party. Discuss with them your eating plans and ask them to help you stick with your plan. If you are attending a buffet meal, have your spouse or friend fill your plate. The less the temptation, the better. Eat slowly and enjoy each bite. When the party tends to be centered around eating, enjoy the party, but don't plan to overstay. The longer you stay, the more food you'll run into. When you are planning your own parties, plan a menu that *you* can eat. Emphasize lower-caloried foods, especially vegetables. Your guests will most likely be delighted at the fresher, healthful foods you are serving.

Packing Lunches

You will be ahead of the game if you can take a few minutes and pack your own lunch for work, for yourself, your spouse, and for your children for school. In fact, pack your own lunches when you are planning a trip to the country or to the beach, or even for a shopping trip. On special occasions you can eat out in restaurants, but considering the limited selection for your diet that you will have at most eating establishments, the loss of time and money involved with eating out and the exposure to foods which although may appeal to you, you'd be better off without, you should bring your own food to eat whenever possible. Yes, it takes effort, planning, and time to pack a lunch, but it's a small and worthwhile investment. The food you pack never has to be boring. Look over the menus in chapter 7 for ideas. "Lunchboxes" are available which are insulated. There are thermoses for hot and cold foods. In these you can include soup, yogurt, cold salads, cheese, milk, or juice. There will be days that you will not have time to comb your hair let alone pack a lunch, so keep an emergency supply of food in your office desk. These might include very small cans of tuna, a jar of crackers (they stay fresher longer this way), small cans of juice, and fruit. You can also keep a jar of dry cereal in your office so that when you are not able to eat breakfast at home, you can have a can of juice from your desk, and just purchase a carton of milk for your cereal. Be sure to keep a can opener, some plastic flatware, bowls, and napkins in your desk.

A packed lunch need not be bulky. You can tuck a cheese sandwich, some vegetables, and a piece of fresh fruit into your briefcase. However, take the 10 to 15 minutes to prepare a tasty and satisfying lunch. You can prepare most things the night before. You can add items such as salad dressing or hot soup in the morning. Keep moist, juicy foods wrapped separately. Sliced tomatoes can be added to the sandwich before eating. Among my favorite lunch staples are cold chicken, tuna salad, bean salads, sourdough, or whole wheat rolls, cheese, and fruit. If you have access to a microwave oven, you can bring leftovers from the previous night's dinner. By packing your own lunch you will know exactly what you are getting in terms of quantity and quality.

Emergency Cupboard

If you have a full and active life, sometimes your activities will take priority to your food shopping or meal planning. For this reason, you should keep an emergency cupboard. The purpose of this cupboard is to supply you with a couple days' worth of food so that you can stay with your diet in case your refrigerator becomes empty before you have time to restock it. Also, if you get a cold or the flu and can't shop, you can have the secure feeling that you won't succumb to malnutrition or starvation. Select canned goods and dry goods for your emergency cupboard which represent each of the food groups. The following is a sample of what you can stock:

Milk Group
   Nonfat dry milk
   Small cans of evaporated lowfat milk

Starch Group
   Dry cereal
   Pasta
   Rice
   Crackers
   Canned and dry beans such as kidney or garbanzo

Meat Group
   Tuna
   Clams
   Boned chicken
   Canned and dry beans

Vegetable Group
   Canned spinach
   Canned green beans
   Canned tomatoes

Fruit Group
   Canned pineapple
   Canned orange juice
   Canned peaches or pears

From these as a basis, you can create breakfast, lunch, and dinner. For example, at breakfast you could have orange juice and oatmeal cooked with the nonfat dry milk. For lunch you could make a minestrone soup with the canned spinach, tomatoes, green beans, and dry beans, with pineapple for dessert. A good dinner could be a clam and rice casserole with a vegetable and a fruit for dessert. While the Alive and Well Diet emphasizes fresh foods, the emergency cupboard will see you through the occasional times when your only alternatives are going out for a fast-food restaurant meal or eating a box of graham crackers. Remember to restock the cupboard as soon as you have used an item from it.

Pregnancy

Because many of the readers of this book are women who might be pregnant one day, a word of caution about dieting. Pregnancy is never the time to follow a weight-reducing diet plan. Maternal weight gain during pregnancy and maternal prepregnancy weight have been found to be the two most influential factors in determining infant birth weight. Infant birth weight bears a very important influence on infant well-being and infant survival. Low birth weight is associated with increased morbidity and mortality. It is thought that one of the reasons why the United States ranks below several other countries in infant survival is due to the fact that U.S. infants have a lower birth weight. These lower weights are partially the result of outdated and erroneous obstetric advice that had women restrict their weight gain to less than 15 pounds. Now the American Medical Association's College of Obstetricians and Gynecologists recommends that women gain between 24 and 27 pounds in the course of their pregnancy. The weight gain should be smooth and start around the third month of pregnancy. The developing fetus has a critical need for essential nutrients. Your baby's physical and mental development and future well-being depend to a great extent on what you eat during pregnancy. If you need to lose weight, do so before planning to become pregnant. During pregnancy you will need to consume a minimum of 4 milk units, 8 meat units, 6 starch units, 3 or more fruit units, and at least 2 vegetable units. Your physician will be able to provide you with more information.

Vegetarian Diets

The Alive and Well Diet can be adjusted for vegetarians who consume milk products and eggs, called lacto-ovo vegetarians. The meat unit list can become the protein unit list to include cheese, eggs, legumes such as dried beans, peas, and lentils, peanut butter, and tofu, all of which are in the old "meat" unit list. For example, for the 3 meat units at dinner, the vegetarian might include 1 cup of cooked beans plus 1 ounce of cheese, or 1 egg and 2 ounces of cheese, and so forth.

Because legumes are an incomplete protein source, the meal in which legumes are consumed should also include a complementary protein source such as a grain or dairy product. A protein is considered an incomplete protein source when it contains one or more of the nine essential amino acids in limited quantities. By combining a protein food source which is low in one or more amino acids with a protein food which possesses that limiting amino acid, but may itself be limited in another amino acid, the two incomplete proteins together make a complete protein source. Each protein is complementary to the other. The two complementary protein sources must be present in the same meal. The body manufactures body proteins for use in tissue and blood cells. In order for this manufacturing to proceed, all necessary amino acids must be present at the same time. An example of two complementary proteins are legumes and grains. Legumes are low in the amino acid methionine, but relatively high in lysine. Grains are low in lysine, but high in methionine. When legumes and grains are combined in a meal, such as pea soup with a wheat roll, the deficiency of one protein is complemented by the other protein. The protein value of the two proteins together is superior to the value of each protein separately. Milk products or eggs when eaten with incomplete protein sources enhance the quality of the protein of the meal.

Because iron requirements for women during the childbearing years are so high, 18 milligrams per day compared to 10 milligrams per day for adult men, female vegetarians will find it especially hard to meet their dietary requirements for iron, and possibly zinc. Both of these minerals are in high concentration in meat. Although these are also present in nonanimal protein sources, the absorption of these minerals is decreased by the presence of phytate found in grains. Phytate binds with iron, zinc, and calcium to form an insoluble product which is not absorbed by the small intestine. Dietary supplementation must often be resorted to. This is especially true when the calories in the diet are restricted. Strict vegetarians who do not consume any animal products need to be very well informed about selecting a diet which provides adequate nutrients. Strict vegetarians are at a risk for consuming diets deficient in iron, zinc, vitamin B_{12}, and calcium. I refer vegetarians to the informative book, *Diet for a Small Planet*, by Francis Lappe, and to *Laurel's Kitchen, A Handbook for Vegetarian Cookery and Nutrition*, by Laurel Robertson, Carol Flinders, and Bronwen Godfrey.

Iron

As discussed, the iron requirements for women of childbearing age are quite high. At 18 milligrams per day recommended dietary allowance, the requirement is almost twice as high as compared with the requirements for the adult male. Women require greater amounts of iron as a result of iron loss in menstrual flow. Although information concerning dietary iron intake is still fragmentary, dietary surveys indicate that the diets of most people in the United States contain about 6 milligrams of iron per 1,000 calories of intake. So, for the "average" diet to reach the recommended 18 milligrams of iron per day, 3,000 calories would have to be consumed daily, unless special dietary iron supplements are provided. Chronic underconsumption of iron can result in iron deficiency anemia. Iron deficiency is the most common deficiency of a nutrient in the world, as well as in the United States. Iron deficiency is common in infants and is nearly universal in the premature infant. Among young healthy women it is estimated that about 50 percent will be iron deficient during some part of their reproductive years. Iron deficiency can result from inadequate diet as well as from blood loss, or from repeated pregnancies, or from any combination of these factors. Iron deficiency anemia decreases level of function and can result in substandard performance. It has been suggested that iron deficiency may produce scholastic underachievement and behavioral disturbances in children. Some individuals with iron deficiency anemia are often unaware of their condition as a result of the slow and gradual development of the anemia. Symptoms associated with iron deficiency anemia are commonly reported to be weakness, fatigue, pallor, shortness of breath upon exertion, rapid heartbeat, and just excessive tiredness.

The amount of iron in the diet as well as the extent of absorption of that iron are equally important factors influencing total iron status. Iron is well absorbed from animal products such as meat, poultry, and fish. Although iron is also found in vegetables, grains, and dairy products, the body does not absorb iron from these sources as readily in the intestinal tract. Certain foods may enhance or hinder iron absorption. Orange juice, or other foods high in vitamin C may double the absorption of iron from a meal, while milk or tea halves the iron absorbed from the same meal. The presence of meat protein such as beef, pork, and poultry in a meal also seems to enhance iron absorption from nonmeat iron sources. Certain cooking utensils may increase the iron content of the food. Cooking in cast-iron skillets can contribute significantly to the iron content of cooked food. The inclusion of high iron foods in the diet several times a week is a sound practice for most women. Liver, beef, lamb, pork, poultry, and cream of wheat cereal, are especially high in iron. The addition of even small quantities of meat protein to meals which are composed of mostly nonmeat sources improves the total iron available from that meal. Among nonanimal sources of iron are dry beans, spinach, and whole grain breads and cereals. Including a high vitamin C food such as citrus fruits or citrus juices in a meal can enhance the absorption of iron from nonanimal iron sources.

10 / Behavioral Modification Approach To Weight Loss

The goal of the Alive and Well Diet is to provide you with enough information so that you will be your own weight loss expert. In the previous chapters, you have learned basic nutritional concepts and definitions. You have learned a categorization system of foods called the food unit lists, that permit you to approximate calorie levels of foods. You have also learned how to prepare food in a lower calorie method. The last chapter discussed how you can manage certain situations arising out of daily living in a way that can help you stay on your diet. Now I will show you other techniques that you can use to alter your behavior to allow you to stay with your goal to reduce your weight. These techniques are behavior modification approaches.

The theory behind the behavior modification approach is that both normal and abnormal behaviors arise and continue from basic learning patterns. These learning principles can be applied to eliminate undesirable behaviors, and to initiate new and better behavior patterns. Inappropriate eating patterns such as overeating, eating high calorie foods, snacking in between meals, and eating too fast, are mostly overlearned habits. Each of the behavioral methods which will be discussed will serve to increase your awareness of what and why you are eating, and to allow you to substitute better habits for the old habits.

Self-Monitoring

A behavioral tool frequently used with much success is self-monitoring. Self-monitoring involves recording the food you eat in the quantities that you eat. Essentially, you need to keep a food diary. Right after you eat a meal, or eat any food item record the food and the quantity that you consume. Look up the approximate calorie value of that food or of the total meal. Figuring the calorie value will be relatively easy when you are carefully following the Alive and Well Diet. The diet plans are planned to be either 1,500 or 1,200 calories. By following the number of food units per meal from either plan, the appropriate calorie level will be reached. Refer to chapter 6 for the food units lists and the calorie value of each list. Recording what you eat will aid you in keeping track of the food units you should be eating. If you indulge in a little extra at one meal, you will have recorded that and be able to reduce your intake later on in the day. Here's an example of a day's entry in the food diary.

Breakfast	Food Units	Calories
½ c orange juice	1 fruit	50
2 slices toast	2 starch	140
2 tsp butter	2 fat	90
coffee	free	
½ c milk	½ milk	70
Lunch		
3 oz tuna, water packed	3 meat	165
2 tsp mayonnaise	2 fat	90
2 slices bread	2 starch	140

Breakfast	Food Units	Calories
vegetable salad	1 vegetable	25
1 tbsp dressing	1 fat	45
1 c milk	1 milk	140
½ melon	2 fruit	100

Dinner		
spaghetti with meat sauce (1 c spaghetti and ½ c meat sauce)	2 starch	140
	2 meat	140
1 c broccoli, steamed	1 vegetable	25
1 slice garlic bread	1 starch	70
1 tsp butter	1 fat	45
½ c orange sherbet		120
	Total Calories	1,595

The ½ cup of sherbet which does not appear in the food lists of chapter 6, is listed among the "Calorie Values of Desserts" in chapter 9. While it is not a regular part of the diet, it is important for you to be aware of the calories it or any other food you eat contains. Many prepared foods have the calories per portion listed on the labels. Booklets of calorie levels of foods are widely available and inexpensive. Calorie charts differ somewhat in the average values for foods listed, but in the course of averaging a number of items, the totals will be similar. From this example of one day's food intake, you can see that it was in excess of 100 calories above the 1,500-calorie level. There were 6 fat units consumed over the course of the day, rather than the 4 on the 1,500-calorie diet plan. There were fewer milk and meat units. So, not only was the calorie intake over 1,500 calories, but there was also deviation in the nutritional composition of the diet. The food diary can be instructive in showing you how many calories you have taken in, and how many calories various foods contain. It will be your daily account. Keeping the diary is particularly useful when you are just starting the Alive and Well Diet and are becoming familiar with the food unit system. Remember to include everything you eat in the diary.

Are there certain times of the day when you are more apt to overeat? Are there any activities that you perform regularly while eating (TV watching, talking on the phone, reading, or studying)? Are there certain foods that you keep overeating that contribute to excessive calorie intake? Maybe you have a weakness for ice cream, or nuts? Are you more apt to overeat when you are with certain people, or when you feel bored, or depressed? There may be certain situations of which you are not yet aware that influence your eating. Your food diary can help you identify these situations. For each meal or for each food that you eat, write down next to it in your food diary the *time* you ate, *where* you ate, *what* you were doing while you ate, *who* you were with, and *how* you were feeling while you were eating. After you have compiled several such expanded food diaries, you might be able to identify a pattern. This self-assessment of your eating habits can help you pinpoint under which situations you are most likely to overeat, and conversely, undereat. Your awareness of these factors is critical. Next, you will see how you can modify your environment to minimize the impact of adverse situations.

Stimulus Control and Environmental Management

Stimulus control and environmental management are two very important behavioral methods that you can use to control your eating. The desire to eat and feelings of hunger occur mostly when the body signals that it is in need of an energy source, food. The signals we are most familiar with are stomach pangs and rumbles. These are internal, physiological stimuli to hunger. There are other stimuli to hunger. Seeing attractive pictures of luscious food, listening to mouth-watering descriptions of food, smelling pleasant food aromas, and even being aware of the hour of the day (12:00 P.M. signals you're ready for lunch) can arouse your desire to eat. These are external stimuli to hunger. Although you may not be physiologically hungry, you eat in response to a strong desire triggered by these powerful external signals. Some researchers have investigated the differences in the influence of external stimuli to eating between the nonoverweight and the overweight. It appears that some overweight people are overly responsive to external stimuli to eat. This presents a real problem for the would-be dieter. Television ads for food, billboards, magazines, and the radio, constantly expose us to temptations. Since the stimuli affect our desire to eat, if we could control or limit our exposure to these stimuli, we could control our eating. The process by which we do this is called environmental management—you change your environment in ways that help you minimize external signals to eat and keep you on your diet.

Minimizing Visual Signals

The sight of food is one of the strongest signals to eat. If the mere sight of a box of candy sitting on the counter encourages you to eat, then getting the candy out of your sight can reduce the temptation to eat it. Sounds simple, but it works. If you can't see it, you probably won't eat it—out of sight, out of mind and mouth. It would be better if those tempting foods were never brought into the home in the first place. However, if other family members must have those foods in the house—cookies, candy, and chips, store them in a hard to reach cupboard, somewhere you would not routinely go. This limits your exposure to troublesome foods. Ask your family not to eat their snack foods in front of you. Similarly, limit your exposure to food at the dinner table by leaving the table as soon as you are finished eating. Watching others who are still eating may encourage you to eat more food. As soon as everyone else has finished eating, arrange to have any leftovers put away immediately. It would be ideal if some other person could perform this task. Again, store the food from the meal in a way that reduces your visual exposure to it. Use opaque plastic containers and store more tempting items behind less troublesome foods. Freezing leftovers provides an obstacle to potential refrigerator raids. If you have been packing lunches for others in your family, ask them, if possible, if they can pack their lunch themselves. Each time you handle food you are exposing yourself to a stimuli which may be too strong to thwart and you might give in. Even a little is too much if it is not on your diet plan.

Remember to jot down everything you eat in your food diary, as well as the time, place, what you were doing, and how you were feeling while you were eating. Calories can add up quickly by just a little bite here and there. When you are reviewing your diary reexamine the association your eating had with how you felt while you were eating, where you were, what time it was, and so forth. If you analyze these carefully you might find that indeed your environment and mood made a difference in your eating.

Disassociate Eating from Other Activity

You need to disassociate eating from any other activity. Do not watch television, read newspapers or magazines, study, or talk on the phone while you eat. When you eat, give eating your full attention. By not doing anything else you won't be eating automatically. You will be concentrating more on tasting your food and appreciating it more. Attempt to consciously slow your rate of eating. Put only one bite of food into your mouth at a time. Put your fork down between bites, chew, and swallow the food before you reach for the fork again. In the middle of your meal, take a short break. Even if you break for just sixty seconds you will provide a chance for your brain's appetite center to pick up signals which your stomach is sending indicating that your appetite is being satisfied. If you eat too quickly the stomach and the brain do not have a chance to communicate.

In addition to disassociating yourself from other activities while eating, keep your eating confined to the same place. Most likely you will pick your kitchen or dining room table. Do all of your eating here only. Do not eat on the sofa, in bed, on the floor, or while standing in the kitchen in front of the refrigerator. You may have been receiving unconscious signals to eat whenever you were sitting on the sofa relaxing with a book, or reading in bed, especially if these associated behaviors were long-standing. By confining your eating to one spot, you will have a chance to think before you put food into your mouth. Also, plan your meals into a daily schedule. Eat at the same time every day. As mentioned earlier, your meals should be four or five hours apart. By keeping to an eating schedule, you will automatically know when you will be eating again. This way you reduce the number of times that you are thinking and deciding about when you are going to eat. If you get hungry in between meals, (five hours is a long time) schedule snacks from food that you have set aside from a previous meal or from a future meal. In other words, rearrange your meals but keep the total number of food units in the day the same.

Substitute Alternate Behaviors for Eating

Your mood may strongly influence your urge to eat. From interpreting your food diary, did you find that you ate in response to feelings of stress, anxiety, tiredness, or boredom? Many overweight people do. While everyone experiences any or all of these feelings throughout the course of the day, you may be trying to manage or control your feelings by eating. This may have developed into an automatic response. By recognizing when these feelings arise, you may be able to intercept them before they lead to eating by substituting alternate behaviors for the eating. Plan an alternate outlet whether it is doing a needed household cleaning chore, exercising to music, giving yourself a manicure and pedicure, reading from a book you enjoy, or anything that distracts you from eating. Choose an activity that will counter your mood, for example, a calming activity when you feel stressed (maybe exercise calms you), a nice hot bath and a nap when you feel tired, a pleasant, luxurious activity when you feel bored. It is important that you become aware of some of the emotions that trigger your eating. If you just feel like eating, for no particular reason other than sheer pleasure, still give yourself something else to do that you can't do if you are eating. Recognize the urge to eat and substitute another pleasant activity in its place.

Self-Control and Motivation

All of the preceding techniques have been tested and proven effective in many studies. They all involve a certain degree of self-control and of motivation. The techniques discussed so far are designed to increase your awareness of your eating and to decrease the risk from temptations without depending solely on "willpower." However, for the techniques to work, you must use them. To start and to continue to use them you need to have motivation to change your behavior as it affects your food consumption. Clearly changing your eating patterns involves hard work on your part. Long-term maintenance of a weight loss depends on your daily behavior and on the decisions you make. You must realize at the onset that *you* are personally responsible for your own behavior and commitment to change. A combination of the best diet and the best techniques in behavior modification will be ineffectual unless you are ready for this commitment of time and effort.

You need to establish realistic goals for yourself. When you make an attainable goal and realize that goal, you set up a chain of positive events, each feeding from the others. Earlier in this book we discussed that the goal of the Alive and Well Diet is a slow and gradual weight loss of about two pounds per week. By its higher calorie content, the Alive and Well Diet will keep most people satisfied physiologically. By the wide variety and selection of foods it contains, most palates will also be satisfied. These features of the diet help you from feeling deprived. The commitment to stop over-eating or eating the wrong foods is difficult enough without adding deprivation into the picture. When you are thinking about your goals, think short-term goals. Eight pounds loss in one month is easier to think about than thirty pounds in four months. Although we have discussed several techniques of behavior modification which you should use, be satisfied if you use just half of them for now. That is a more realistic goal than expecting to alter all your food-related behavior at the same time.

Positive Reinforcement and Social Support

Sticking to a diet is difficult, even when the diet is a highly nutritious, nondeprivational diet, such as the Alive and Well Diet. If the diet represents a major change from your old, accustomed eating patterns, you may have difficulty in not returning to your old habits. It takes a genuine effort to change old habits, especially eating habits. The rewards for sticking to your diet and losing weight are not immediate. They are future rewards. When you eat something delicious, the good taste is the immediate gratification. For most of us, the immediate gratification is more powerful than the patient anticipation of future rewards.

One way to increase your ability to stick with your diet is to reward yourself. Plan in advance how you will reward yourself when you meet one of your short-term goals. Your reward, of course, should not be food. It can be an article of clothing, a visit to a beauty salon for a facial, a small piece of jewelry, anything that you consider a treat. In the beginning of your weight loss, most of your positive reinforcement will be coming directly from you. Other people may not notice your progress early on during your weight loss, and might be reluctant to comment on your appearance anyway.

Experience has shown that positive reinforcement and social support can be very helpful for dieters. Try your family first. Ask yourself if yours is a family which can provide you with the help and support you'll need. Not all families can. Some families may resent the change in life-style and routine that they foresee your diet might impose on them. If you feel that your family has the potential to help you, ask them. They will need to understand how they can be most helpful. Explain to them about your diet and what you will be eating. They will want to know how things will be different. Ask them to help you by snacking away from you. Ask them to help keep foods out of sight, clear off the table, put food away, and help themselves to food instead of asking you for it. When you do the shopping, tell your family that you will not be able to buy foods that are incompatible with your diet such as chips, sodas, and pastry. Ask them to buy these foods, if they want them, themselves. Prepare the family's food as for your own diet. It will be a more healthful diet for them also, as well as a preventive measure. Encourage family members to participate in exercise with you. Go walking together, ride bikes, play tennis. Your husband or older children can help you review your food diary. You may also wish to keep a chart of your progressive weight loss so that your family can see it. By involving them in this way they can provide you with the encouragement and congratulations you require.

You may be able to receive support from your friends. If you have a close friend with whom you feel comfortable to discuss your diet, try it. Tell her that she could help you by limiting your exposure to food when you are together. Discuss participating less in food-related social activities. If you have a friend who also desires to lose weight, ask if she would be interested in starting the Alive and Well Diet with you. Discuss your progress together. Listen to each other's problems and suggestions. Take up an activity program together.

Life-style Changes

As we have been saying since the beginning of this book, the goal of the Alive and Well Diet is the long-term maintenance of weight loss. Long-term mainte-nance depends on long-term changes in eating behaviors. The behavior modification tools just discussed can help you in changing from your old patterns. For you to maintain your desired weight level it is necessary for you to adopt more healthful life-style changes which include a more nutritious diet permanently and more physical activity. It may be necessary for your entire family to adopt these life-style changes in order to effectively maintain healthy weight levels.

11 / Exercise: A Critical Ingredient in a Weight Loss Program

No program geared for weight reduction can be considered complete without an exercise component. The lack of sufficient activity accounts for most of the increasing incidence of overweight in the United States. Today, in the United States, we consume approximately ten percent fewer calories each day than our ancestors ate at the turn of this century. Since then, the percentage of overweight people in the United States has doubled. The obvious reason is that today, our activity is far less than what it was in 1900. In work and at home, mechanization has replaced much of the work that in earlier times was done with physical effort. If you were to add up all the calories that you would spend each day in performing certain tasks yourself, rather than depending on machines, you would get a significant number of calories. These calories our ancestors spent daily. These same calories represent what we convert to fat, since our activity is much lower. The gradual weight gain that comes with middle age is usually *not* as a result of eating more than when one was in high school or college. The big difference is less physical activity with increasing age. Weight gain occurs when eating habits do not change in relation to decreasing physical activity. At very sedentary levels, calorie requirements are so low that hunger would be a lifelong problem for most individuals desiring to stay trim. It is easier to build into your life an exercise program than it is to chronically deprive yourself of food. The Alive and Well Diet which is intended to form the foundation of a lifelong healthful eating style works best with an exercise component.

There are two main reasons why you should exercise. One is to lose weight, the other is to improve your cardiovascular system. First, with respect to weight loss, you don't have to change your daily routine by very much in order to burn more calories. Increasing the number of steps you take daily by walking where you formerly would drive and climbing stairs where you formerly took an elevator, can add up your calorie expenditure. Even small amounts of exercise scattered throughout the day, such as 10 minutes of exercise before going to work in the morning, and 10 minutes before bedtime are effective in helping you lose weight. Make it a habit to incorporate as much activity into your daily living as possible. By just including a half hour walk into your day's routine, you can shed 12 pounds in a year and not even change your calorie intake.

Ideally, the exercise program you follow for fat loss should be one to improve cardiovascular function. This type of activity is also the most effective for weight loss. The term that is used to distinguish this type of exercise from the other forms of exercises is *aerobic*. Aerobic, as the word would indicate, refers to the type of activity which consumes large amounts of *air*, specifically oxygen. When you are engaged in aerobic exercise, you are breathing harder, your heart beats faster, and you perspire. For cardiovascular changes to come about, an individual has to work between 70 and 80 percent of his maximum heart rate and sustain that rate for at least 20 minutes. The heart, as a result of this training, develops into a stronger muscle which is able to pump out more blood with each beat. Your resting heart rate will eventually slow, as a result of a more efficient heart. Although other forms of exercise also result in an increased calorie expenditure, they do not have the same effect on the cardiovascular system. Aerobic exercise is sustained, relatively strenuous activity which works the heart and lungs, and which utilizes a greater percentage of fat as fuel as compared with nonaerobic exercise.

Exercise has other benefits besides contributing to weight loss and cardiovascular fitness. Regular exercise, as discussed earlier in the book, actually helps to control appetite. Appetite does not increase with exercise. The appetite control center needs a certain amount of exercise to function properly. Studies have shown that in individuals who exercise strenuously for 30 minutes or more per day, the appetite and food intake adjust resulting in a leaner body than in the sedentary state. Appetite increases only after a certain degree of leanness has been achieved. This appears to be a consistent finding in people and in animals.

Regular exercise results in a change in body composition, so that there is a greater lean body mass, and less fatty tissue. Middle-age spread is mostly due to the increased deposit of fat in areas that were formerly muscle. Exercise has a fat store mobilizing effect as a result of the hormonal response to exercise. With exercise not only are fat stores utilized as an energy source, but the deposition of new fat stores is not favored. The increase in lean body tissue, muscle, which exercise brings at the expense of body fat, helps increase strength and endurance. The more strength you build, the fitter you become, and the more you'll feel like engaging in activity.

The change in body composition that results from exercise will increase your basal and resting metabolic rate (BMR), the rate at which your body uses energy, calories. Lean tissue has a greater metabolic rate than fatty tissue, as it is more metabolically active. As your percentage of lean body weight increases in relation to your fat body weight, your BMR will increase correspondingly. This means of course that you will be burning calories at a faster rate even while you are sleeping.

The calorie expenditure of exercise depends on your level of fitness to start with, your present weight, and the duration and intensity of the activity. The more fit you are, the more calories you will burn per minute of that activity. As you progress gradually with your exercise program, all exercise will be more effective for you in terms of the calories expended. Part of this is related to the increased efficiency with which your body can use oxygen when you are more fit. Conversely, the more you weigh, the more energy you will use in your movements. It is as though you were exercising with weights attached to your body. At 180 pounds you will spend more calories in running half a mile than if you weighed 130 pounds. So, if you are overweight, exercise can be even more effective for you. Unfortunately, the heavier you are, the less fit you are, the less likely that you will feel like sustaining activity long enough or often enough to be beneficial to you. The duration of an activity is directly related to the amount of energy expended. Twice as many jumping jacks burns twice as many calories. However, for purposes of calorie expenditure, it doesn't matter if you exercise for 10 minutes three times a day, or for 30 minutes once a day. The total calories spent will be the same. There will be a difference in the effect the exercise has on the cardiovascular system. An activity must be intense enough and of sustained duration, as previously discussed, to improve cardiovascular fitness.

Exercise brings other benefits along with weight loss and improved physical fitness. As the ancient Greeks said, "A sound mind dwells in a sound body." Exercise increases your sense of well-being. You can't help feeling better about yourself with your improving fitness and strength. Chances are, you'll feel less tired at the end of a busy day and you'll have greater tolerance to the stresses of everyday life.

Now that you're sold on the idea of exercise, how should you begin, and with what form of exercise? First and foremost, whenever you change your activity patterns check with your physician. For some individuals who have very low levels of activity, a sudden increase may be too stressful for the body. Your physician can evaluate how much and how quickly you should proceed.

Your goal is to include at least 30 minutes of exercise in your daily routine. Toward the improvement of your cardiovascular system, it would be better if the 30 minutes of activity was concentrated into one intensive activity period. Throughout the rest of the day, increase your routine daily activity by walking more, taking the stairs, and anything else that keeps you moving. The specific type of activity that you select depends on what you like; but remember that for maximum benefit, an activity must be one that keeps you in constant movement for the duration of the exercise period. There should not be periods of rest or inactivity within the exercise, like what you would get while playing golf or bowling or volleyball. Exercise such as walking at a fast pace, swimming, calisthenics involving major muscles and done in continuous succession, riding a stationary bicycle, and jogging, are good examples of activities that burn the most calories and work out the cardiovascular system. A fast game of singles tennis, racquetball, skating, and dancing can also be aerobic in nature. For most people, I find that the easiest way to include a daily activity component is to perform calisthenics in the comfort of their home. Calisthenics can take various forms, from a continuous running pace through the basic calisthenics you probably did in elementary and junior high school, to more dance-influenced "jazzercise" done to music. If you have not exercised for quite awhile, you will need two things: to increase your flexibility by regular stretching, and to reeducation as to good basic exercises. There are a number of programs on TV which can instruct you on how to do basic exercise. As you increase your flexibility and strength, you will be able to do more. Starting slow and easy is very important. If you overdo it in the beginning and get too sore, you will feel less like continuing. Even a 10-minute slow stretch for the first week you start on an exercise program is very acceptable. Work up slowly adding 5 to 10 minutes each week until you reach 30 minutes. All exercise should be preceded by a warm-up stretch to slowly start your heart rate increase, and to bring blood to the muscles which will be worked. Later, as you progress to more intensive activity, you will need a cool-down period where you gradually slow your movements before completely stopping.

I want to caution you about advertisements you will see for devices, creams, lotions, pills, wraps, and more, that claim will reduce you in certain spots by melting the fat away. You cannot reduce in certain spots, the thighs, or abdomen for example. When you restrict your calories by going on a diet, you gradually use the fat stored *throughout* your body for an energy source. When you add exercise, even more of the stored fat is used throughout your body. No particular area of stored fat is used in greater proportion than another area. Exercising leads to a general loss of body fat. By exercising the thigh or abdominal muscles, you will not speed up the loss of fat in that area. However, you will improve the muscle tone in that area which, along with the general fat loss, will improve your appearance. Another word of advice. Do you say to yourself that if only you had the time, or the means, to belong to a health club or spa you would have it made? Health clubs and spas usually have a wide assortment of services, ranging from heavy exercise machines to passive exercise gadgets, to whirlpools, massages, and saunas. Except for the possible benefits that a few of the exercise machines have on improving your muscular strength and on increasing your calorie expenditure, most of the other devices do little more for you than make you feel as if you have accomplished something. Some of the best exercise that you can get you can do in your own home. If you enjoy walking or jogging, you can do this for free in your own neighborhood. If you like swimming, and do not have your own pool, you might consider joining the Y or check with local colleges or the Department of Parks and Recreation. Whatever you choose do it and do it regularly!

The following table shows you the approximate number of calories that you expend when you engage in various activities. Because the number of calories used depends on body weight as well as on the type of activity, calorie levels are provided for in terms of calories per pound of body weight. Bear in mind that not only do you expend the calories listed when you exercise, but that you increase your expenditure of calories even while you sleep by the effect exercise has in increasing your metabolic rate.

ENERGY COST OF ACTIVITIES

Activity	Calories/lb/hour
Aerobic calisthenics	3.1–3.7
Bicycling (moderate speed)	1.1
Dancing (jazz, rock)	1.7
Running or jogging, moderate pace	3.2–6.5
Skating	1.6
Swimming (2 mph)	3.6
Tennis, singles	2.8
Walking (3 mph)	0.91

Note: The above energy costs are exclusive of the calories used in basal metabolism. There will be wide variability in the above values depending on the intensity of exercise and the fitness of the individual.

Calculation of Calories Expended
Example: body weight—150 lbs
swimming—30 minutes
3.6 x 150 x ½ hour = 270 calories expended

12 / Other Diets: You Compare

No doubt, many new "diets" will be appearing, as they always do, in the coming months and years. Currently there are several "diets" which are enjoying a wide popularity. Some of these diets are new, and some are old, recycled diets presented as being new, breakthrough plans. Unfortunately, few of them are based on scientific principles. While most of the popular diets can lead to immediate weight loss because they are low in calories, they may be deficient in essential nutrients. Some may result in undesirable side effects which are detrimental to good health. Actual symptoms of malnutrition may appear after the chronic use of some of the diets, including some of the diets we will be discussing. For example, low protein diets can be particularly harmful, resulting in hair loss, fatigue, and muscle wasting. Low carbohydrate diets can disrupt the acid-base balance of the body leading to a condition known as ketosis, which poses a major concern for those individuals with, or predisposed to, diabetes. In addition, this type of diet can give rise to high uric acid levels which may precipitate kidney stone formation. In the following section, nine of the currently most popular diets will be reviewed.

As it is one of the goals of this book to increase your knowledge of nutrition, at the end of the presentation of these diets, I will review for you what you should look for in a diet plan. You should be able to assess for yourself in the future the adequacy of new, fad diets.

The Atkins Diet

The Atkins Diet is a low carbohydrate, high fat, high protein regimen. This approach yields temporary fast weight loss due to the fact that the body excretes large amounts of water when it has only protein and fat to use for energy. As soon as the diet is stopped, weight is regained as a result of the normal rehydration of body tissues when carbohydrates are eaten again. This diet is nutritionally unbalanced and potentially danger-ous for the following reasons. First, the high fat nature of the diet can raise the levels of cholesterol in the blood and speed up the development of atherosclerosis. Also, high protein intake can lead to an increase in the blood level of uric acid which can precipitate gouty arthritis. When a diet is deficient in carbohydrates, such as in the Atkins Diet, fat is burned for energy which results in the production of toxic substances called ketone bodies. When ketones accumulate in the blood, the condition is called ketosis; the symptoms are nausea, fatigue, dizziness, and general malaise. Excessive pro-tein is stressful to the kidneys which have to work extra hard to get rid of the by-products of protein breakdown. Diets high in protein also cause the body to lose calcium from the bones. The Atkins Diet is low in calcium, vitamins A and C, thiamin, riboflavin, niacin, and fiber. The plan does nothing to encourage lifelong healthful eating patterns.

The Beverly Hills Diet

The Beverly Hills Diet is among the newcomers to the "fad" diet group. Based largely on the consumption of specific fruits with smaller amounts of starches, vegetables, and proteins, this diet purports that fruits, especially tropical fruits, contain high concentrations of enzymes which help to "digest" other foods. The theory is that by combining fresh foods, which allegedly have the magical enzymes, with other foods, proper digestion is ensured and food cannot get "stuck" in the body and turn into fat. This diet is grossly inaccurate in describing the physiological process of digestion, fat metabolism, and in describing the nutritional value of certain foods. As all fruit is very low in protein content, this diet is dangerously low in protein, supplying less than a third of the normal requirement. When protein intake is restricted to intakes lower than that required by the body, muscle tissues are broken down to supply protein for vital organ function. The diet, due to the very narrow variety of foods, is deficient in other nutrients as well, specifically niacin, riboflavin, calcium, iron, and zinc, just to name a few. It is possible to see a weight loss on this diet due to the fact that calories are reduced, and due to water loss from the diarrhea that this diet produces. The diet cannot be followed on a long-term basis and does nothing to instruct you in healthful eating practices. In short, this diet advocates a dangerous approach to weight loss.

The Cambridge Diet

This diet is actually a food substance which is intended to replace one or more or all meals. It is composed of protein, some carbohydrate, fat, vitamins, minerals, and electrolytes. Total calorie content is very low. When the product is taken as the sole source of energy, it provides a little more than 300 calories per day. The Cambridge Diet is based on the protein-sparing modified fast concept. Specifically, this concept is one of a near starvation regimen in which the few calories which are provided are from protein. This protein is intended to provide the body with its daily need for amino acids, the building blocks of protein. This should theoretically reduce or "spare" the body from breaking down its own protein, lean muscle tissue, and increase the proportion of weight loss due to fatty tissue. In actuality, the extent to which lean tissue is spared in this modified fast is still the subject of research. It appears, however, that protein-sparing techniques are more effective in the very overweight (greater than 50 pounds overweight) than in the moderately overweight. It is clear that this approach, as any near-starvation regimen, possesses a great health risk. Under the constant and competent monitor of physicians, the modified fast has been used by some medical centers to reduce morbidly overweight individuals in which the risks posed by the overweight outweigh the risks posed by the diet. But to emphasize, these individuals were under the care of experts, and were for the most part 50 or more pounds overweight. For any weight loss to be long lasting, the individual must learn and develop sound eating habits. A diet such as the Cambridge plan taken alone does not provide a foundation for such learning to take place as real food is not used. Once the diet is discontinued, the dieter is left without guidelines as to how to proceed. The Cambridge Diet Plan uses Cambridge counselors whose only qualifications are that they have lost weight with the diet themselves, and that they attend a few meetings on product updating. This is definitely not a diet plan for anyone to undertake without the strictist of medical supervision. It is a plan reserved only for grossly overweight individuals for whom weight loss is an urgent health concern.

Cellulite

There are many who advocate that a specific diet, a cream, a massage, or a wrap, among other devices, are useful in eliminating cellulite. Cellulite has been described in popular literature as being the result of the accumulation of waste products, toxins, or any other pollutants in the body. We are led to believe that this form of fat is somehow different than other fat in the body. In actuality, there is no scientific basis for distinguishing what has been called cellulite from any other type of body fat. The dimpled appearance of the fat located on the thighs, upper arms, hips, and buttocks of some individuals is due to excessive fat deposits in general, poor muscle tone, and loss of tissue elasticity that occurs with the aging process. The first two, however, excessive fat deposits and poor muscle tone, can best be attacked by decreasing calorie intake and by increasing exercise, particularly aerobic which leads to reduced total body fat. The other devices for helping to rid your body of cellulite will only help to rid you of your money.

The Complete Scarsdale Medical Diet

This diet plan is a high protein, reduced carbohydrate diet, a new variation of an idea that has been around before. These type of diets tend to result in an initially very rapid weight loss as a result of fluid loss, which, once normal carbohydrate intake is resumed, is quickly replaced. The diet does not specify exact amounts of foods; thus the total calorie intake can change daily. Furthermore, there are no milk group products on the diet resulting in low calcium levels in the diet. The diet does not provide a basis for healthful eating once weight loss goals are reached. In the book, the information regarding the dietary treatment of common medical problems is oversimplified and outdated. The Scarsdale Diet, and other diets on the same theme are not recommended.

The I Love New York Diet

This diet book reached best-seller status quickly, and soon faded away. The diet promises a quick initial weight loss of ten pounds in seven days. While the diet offers a variety of foods, the menus prescribed are highly specified. Dieters are not taught how to calculate menus and calories themselves. Rather, rigid and mechanical adherence to the dietary protocol, without involving decision making, is encouraged. Portion sizes are not discussed; rather "restaurant" size portions are advised. Worse yet, a system of alternating a week of a crash diet of inadequate nutritional value with a week of "holiday" eating is one of the major precepts of the diet. Besides imposing physiological stress, this practice does not foster sound eating patterns. Some of the ideas in the diet, such as including foods from the various food groups which unfortunately appears only in the "holiday" eating, and providing lowfat recipes, make this diet somewhat of an improvement over some of the other fad diets. However, the reader of The I Love New York Diet is left with little information as to how to go about keeping weight off, if in fact the diet helps at all in taking weight off.

The Pritikin Program for Diet and Exercise

The Pritikin program's basic diet, the Maintenance Diet, is a dietary plan which together with the program's exercise plan claims to prevent the onset of, or reverse the degenerative diseases such as cardiovascular disease, adult onset diabetes, and certain intestinal disorders. The diet itself is very low in fat, 5 to 10 percent, low in protein, 10 to 15 percent, and high in carbohydrates, about 80 percent. It has been demonstrated by other researchers that indeed, blood cholesterol, blood sugar, and blood pressure can be lowered by a combination of a lower calorie, low fat, low salt, and high starch diet, especially when an exercise component is included. However, a diet as low in animal protein and as high in plant food sources as the Pritikin Maintenance Diet can be marginal in mineral content, especially iron, calcium, zinc, and copper. As mentioned before, plant sources of these nutrients are less well absorbed than animal sources. Another potential problem with the diet is that no guidance is given for correctly combining plant protein foods to insure adequate and complete protein intake. In general, the main points emphasized in the diet—reducing total fat, salt, sugar, and alcohol—have raised the level of consciousness of the public of the relationship between diet, exercise, and good health. However, the recommendations made have been taken to the extreme, and I believe that few can follow the diet as it is prescribed for an extended period of time. The Maximum Weight Loss Diet, a variation of the Maintenance Diet, is very low in total calories and protein, as well as in the B vitamins, iron, and calcium.

Richard Simmons' Never Say Diet Book

The nutrition part of the book does not adequately cover the subject, but most of what Richard Simmons has to say in the book and on TV is accurate. The tips on how to eat, what to eat, and how to prepare food are both informative and entertaining. The nutritional advice is useful, but most overweight people need more information such as portion size, calorie values, and sample menu plans. Richard Simmons has provided an increased awareness for his book readers and TV viewers of the importance of exercise in general well-being and in weight control, and of the importance of taking control of your own health destiny.

The Weight Watchers Program

The program that Weight Watchers International, Inc. has put together over the past years has provided a sensible weight reduction plan for thousands. The program includes a well-balanced diet based on a variety of foods, nutrition and behavioral education, an exercise component, a maintenance plan, as well as group support. To receive the information on the diet, behavior modification, exercise, and so forth, the potential dieter has to become a paid member and attend regular meetings. For some dieters, the expense, effort to attend the meetings, and the group environment are not worth it. For others, it is. The Weight Watchers weight-reducing diet plans are based on 1,200 calories for women, and 1,600 calories for men. These levels might be too low for many dieters to maintain without the constant reinforcement and encouragement of a group situation. In general, the package that Weight Watchers offers incorporates the basic principles that a good weight reduction program should have—a well-balanced diet, a focus on nutrition education and behavior reeducation, and exercise.

Conclusion

As you read or hear about other "new" diets in the future, you will be able to assess their nutritional adequacy based on the knowledge that you have acquired through this book. Compare the "new" diet's recommended meal plan against the Basic Four Food Groups, and the dietary guidelines discussed in chapter 5. If the diet falls below the minimum recommended levels and does not follow the dietary guidelines, chances are that it is not nutritionally sound. A diet offering a "quick" weight loss is to be questioned as fat can only be lost at the rate of 1 to 2 pounds per week. Weight loss in excess of this will be largely from lean body tissue and water. A diet which falls below 1,200 calories will almost always be lacking in important nutrients. To be most effective in weight control, a diet must provide a means of education for the dieter so that a life-style of healthful eating will be continued once weight loss has occurred. Lastly, but very importantly, a weight-reducing diet should incorporate an exercise component for maximum effectiveness. It shouldn't come as a surprise that the Alive and Well Diet incorporates all of these principles.

13 / Reaching Your Weight Goal

The laws of nature dictate that when calorie intake falls below energy needs, weight will be lost. You will reach your weight goal by staying with your diet and by following an exercise program. When you reach your goal, *congratulations*! That was a lot of hard work, but you did it! Now what? Can you go back to the way you ate before you started the diet? Can you let loose of the reins? I know that you know the answer. Since the beginning of this book, I have said that the biggest problem for the overweight is not weight loss, but weight maintenance. Statistics show that the majority of individuals who are successful in weight loss eventually put the weight back on. The reason is a return to former poor eating habits which caused the increased weight in the first place. The diets that caused the weight loss were not diets that created a permanent change in eating patterns. Behavioral changes such as eating patterns are facilitated by practice. By the time you have reached your weight goal on the Alive and Well Diet, you will have had sufficient practice in the new, desirable eating pattern. After your weight loss, the eating pattern that you follow will be similar to your weight-reducing plan except that total calories will be increased. Now, I can hear many of you moaning, will you have to be "on a diet" for the rest of your life? In the sense that a program of nutritious, sensible, and enjoyable eating is a diet, yes. You have to be conscious of what you are eating, always, even when the excess weight is off. I can almost guarantee you that if you do not, you will be right back to your old weight. You can splurge occasionally when you are maintaining your weight, but not on a routine basis.

The term *diet* has recently lost favor with some weight loss "experts." It is no longer fashionable to speak of "diets" for weight loss. Some will tell you that "diets" don't work and aren't the answer. After an analysis of some of the popular "diets" currently making the rounds, it is evident that the "diets" weren't the answer. We have been saying all along that your *diet*—and I use that term in its true denotation, that is, what a person usually eats or drinks—must be a *lifelong* plan of healthful eating. It is not something you go "off" when your weight goals are realized. Along with eating habit changes, changes in the way you think of food and in the way you feel about yourself must also be made. Physical exercise also needs to be included in a complete weight control program. Diet cannot be isolated as the only factor involved in weight reduction. The Alive and Well Diet encompasses all the variables that are involved in weight control. In this sense it is more of a life-style program than a *diet* in the popular sense of the word.

The good news is that you will be able to increase your total calorie intake by several hundred calories by increasing the quantities of the various food unit groups. As reviewed in chapter 3, you can calculate the approximate number of calories that you need to maintain your weight by multiplying your present weight by a factor of from 12 to 18 calories per pound, based on your activity and age. This approximate level of calorie requirements is a guide, a starting point. Weigh yourself daily to see if your weight has changed up or downward so that you can adjust your eating accordingly. With this guide, you will select the appropriate basic plan to follow. The following diet plans are based on the same principles as the reducing plans. They include a wide variety of foods to assure adequate intake of all essential nutrients, are low in fat, high in complex carbohydrates, high in fruits and vegetables, moderate in protein, and low in sugar and salt.

1,800-Calorie Basic Plan

Breakfast
  2 fruit units
  2 starch units
  2 fat units
  1 milk unit

Lunch
  3 meat units
  3 starch units
  2 fat units
  vegetable units as desired
  1 milk unit
  1 fruit unit

Dinner
  3 meat units
  3 starch units
  2 fat units
  vegetable units as desired
  1 milk unit
  2 fruit units

2,000-Calorie Basic Plan

Use 1,800-plan, adding:
  1 milk unit
  1 fruit unit

2,200-Calorie Basic Plan

Use 1,800-plan, adding:
  1 milk unit
  1 fruit unit
  1 starch unit
  1 meat unit
  1 fat unit

The additional food units may be added at any of the meals or may be used as a snack. The 1,800-Calorie

Basic Plan can be a weight-reducing plan for a large man, or for a physically active man. The 2,200-Calorie Plan is included as a maintenance plan for physically active women, or moderately active men of smaller stature. If you calculate that you require more calories than 2,200, increase all food units by a small amount until you establish by checking on your scale what level maintains your weight.

When you are at your weight goal, you won't have to be compulsive about everything you eat, but you will need to be aware of the quantities and of the types of foods you are eating. The more familiar you become with the food unit system, which is a convenient way to keep track of total calorie intake, the easier it will be for you to maintain your weight. You can adjust the diet plan for special occasions when you want to indulge in things you usually don't. Keep exercising. This keeps you feeling good physically and mentally. It keeps your appetite in check and keeps your proportion of lean body mass to fat body mass high.

I hope that through this book that you have acquired a great deal more knowledge about nutrition and weight control. I hope that you will continue to apply this new information. Old habits do die hard, and only your desire and motivation can make you permanently change your old habits. You have that desire, and maybe all at once, or through a series of small steps, you will do it. The main thing is that you know that you can take responsibility for improving and maintaining your life and well-being. Good luck to you.

Index

ABOUT THE AUTHOR

Diane Jouganatos has been with the *Alive and Well* television show since the spring of 1982. She brings to the show a strong background in nutrition. She received a Bachelor of Science degree in Dietetics and Nutrition from the University of California at Davis, and a Master in Public Health Nutrition from the University of California at Los Angeles, and completed a dietetic internship at the Wadsworth Veterans Administration Hospital. She's a member of the American Dietetic Association and has worked as a clinical nutritionist at the Women's Hospital of Los Angeles County-University of Southern California Medical Center, and at the UCLA Medical Center. Ms. Jouganatos has lectured before professional and community groups and is currently in private practice in Santa Monica, California. She combines a rich scientific background in nutrition with a love of good food in her new approach to eating and cooking.

NEED MORE INFORMATION ON YOUR HEALTH AND NUTRITION?

Read the books that will lead you to
a happier and healthier life.

☐	05024	THE JAMES COCO DIET James Coco & Marion Paone (A Hardcover Book)	$13.95
☐	23888	ARTHRITIC'S COOKBOOK Dong & Bank	$3.50
☐	20925	WHAT'S IN WHAT YOU EAT Will Eisner	$3.95
☐	34106	MY BODY, MY HEALTH Stewart & Hatcher (A Large Format Book)	$11.95
☐	22872	WOMEN AND THE CRISES IN SEX HORMONES G. Seamans	$4.50
☐	22673	CONCISE MEDICAL DICTIONARY Laurance Urdange Associates	$4.95
☐	23335	GH-3-WILL IT KEEP YOU YOUNG LONGER H. Bailey	$3.95
☐	23827	THE HERB BOOK J. Lust	$4.95
☐	23767	HOPE AND HELP FOR YOUR NERVES C. Weekes	$3.95
☐	23818	PEACE FROM NERVOUS SUFFERING C. Weekes	$3.95
☐	24279	SIMPLE, EFFECTIVE TREATMENT OF AGORAPHOBIA C. Weekes	$3.95

Prices and availability subject to change without notice.